AUJESZKY'S DISEASE

CURRENT TOPICS IN VETERINARY MEDICINE AND ANIMAL SCIENCE

VOLUME 17

AUJESZKY'S DISEASE

A Seminar in the Animal Pathology Series
of the CEC Programme of Coordination of
Agricultural Research, held at
Tübingen, Federal Republic of Germany
June 9-10, 1981

Sponsored by the Commission of the European Communities,
Directorate-General for Agriculture, Coordination of
Agricultural Research

Edited by

G. Wittmann
Bundesforschungsanstalt für
Viruskrankheiten der Tiere
Tübingen, Federal Republic of Germany.

S.A. Hall
Ministry of Agriculture, Fisheries & Food
London, United Kingdom.

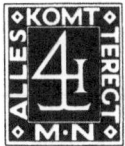

1982

MARTINUS NIJHOFF PUBLISHERS
THE HAGUE / BOSTON / LONDON

for

THE COMMISSION OF THE EUROPEAN COMMUNITIES

Distributors

for the United States and Canada
Kluwer Boston, Inc.
190 Old Derby Street
Hingham, MA 02043
USA

for all other countries
Kluwer Academic Publishers Group
Distribution Center
P.O. Box 322
3300 AH Dordrecht
The Netherlands

Library of Congress Cataloging in Publication Data
Main entry under title:

Aujeszky's disease.

   (Current topics in veterinary medicine and animal science ; 17)
   1. Pseurorabies--Congresses. I. Wittmann, G.
(Günther), 1926-   . II. Hall, S. A.
III. Commission of the European Communities.
Directorate-General for Agriculture. Coordination
of Agricultural Research. IV. Series. [DNLM:
1. Pseudorabies--Congresses. 2. Pseudorabies
virus--Congresses. W1 CU822B v. 17 / SF 809.P8
A923 1981]

SF809.P8A93   636.089'659   82-2173
ISBN-13:978-94-009-7555-2   AACR2

ISBN-13:978-94-009-7555-2   e-ISBN-13:978-94-009-7553-8
DOI: 10.1007/978-94-009-7553-8

Publication arranged by
Commission of the European Communities,
Directorate-General Information Market and Innovation

EUR 7638 EN

© ECSC, EEC, EAEC, Brussels-Luxemburg, 1982
Softcover reprint of the hardcover 1st edition 1982

Manuscript Preparation by
Janssen Services, 33a High Street, Chislehurst, Kent BR7 5AE, UK

LEGAL NOTICE

Neither the Commission of the European Communities nor any person acting on behalf of the Commission is responsible for the use which might be made of the following information.

CONTENTS

.

PREFACE

Aujeszky's disease (AD) is increasing in Europe and it has become a serious problem in some of the countries of the European Communities (EC). The control and eradication of the disease is very difficult since AD virus (ADV) evokes a persistant latent infection in its main host, the pig. Such latent infection can also occur when vaccinated pigs are exposed to the virus.

In view of this, the Commission of the European Communities (CEC) thought it necessary to have a survey on the current state of knowledge on AD and ADV. Therefore, a seminar was organised by the Federal Research Institute for Animal Virus Diseases in Tübingen, Federal Republic of Germany, and held there on June 9 and 10, 1981. The seminar was a part of the 'Animal Pathology Programme' of the CEC. The seminar was attended by 44 participants from the countries of the EC, and 29 papers were presented which covered a wide field of research on AD: properties of the virus, diagnostic procedures, immunity and pathogenesis, vaccination, latent infection, epidemiology, control and eradication. Scientists from different institutes in the EC who have been working on AD thus had the opportunity to exchange their knowledge as well as to give and receive impetus for further scientific work. Furthermore, many details were given which are of interest for the veterinary authorities with regard to control and eradication of AD.

I would like to take this opportunity of thanking all those who contributed to the success of the seminar. I want to mention the excellent work of Janssen Services for the preparation of the Proceedings. Last, but not least, I thank the CEC for financing this seminar and   J. Connell from the CEC for his support.

G. Wittmann

INTRODUCTION

AUJESZKY'S DISEASE

G. Wittmann

Federal Research Institute for Animal Virus Diseases,
D-7400 Tübingen, Federal Republic of Germany.

Aujeszky's disease (AD) has been known for about 150 years. The disease is characterised by encephalomyelitis and, in conjunction with this, the naso-pharyngeal, tracheal and pulmonary regions are frequently affected.

AD is caused by a DNA virus of about 180 nm in size with a very complex protein structure. The virus belongs to the herpes virus group. Some antigenic relationship exists between Aujeszky's disease virus (ADV) and other members of the group.

ADV is fairly resistant to high temperatures and very resistant to acid and alkaline pH. Therefore, the virus can persist in the natural environment for several weeks. Chemicals that cleave off chlorine are the most effective disinfectants. Formalin is second choice. Sodium hydroxide is unsuitable.

Pigs are the primary host of the virus although a large number of other species can be infected naturally or experimentally. The most important of these are cattle, sheep, goats, dogs, cats and foxes on fur farms. Primates, solipeds and birds are highly resistant. Natural infection occurs via the nasal and oral routes but the virus can also enter the body by way of the vagina and foetuses can become infected in the uterus. In pigs the morbidity and the mortality rates are dependent on the age of the animals and because they decrease with rising age, piglets and young pigs are most at risk from the disease. With other species the course of infection is usually lethal and recovery is an exception.

The clinical symptoms in pigs are, on the one hand, those evoked by the effect on the central nervous system (CNS) such as loss of voice, disorder of movement, tremor, convulsions, paralysis and somnolence. On the other hand, there can be symptoms caused by the respiratory tract being affected; nasal discharge, coughing, and pneumonia. In other species there may, in addition, be pruritus. Maceration of the foetuses and still-birth is often observed after ADV infection of pregnant sows.

Primary virus multiplication takes place in the cells of the naso-pharyngeal region and of the respiratory tract. From these places the virus invades the CNS by the neural pathway. The virus is also disseminated throughout the body to different organs and tissues in pigs by the leukocytes in blood and lymph.

The virus is excreted in nasal, vaginal and preputial secretions and in the milk.

ADV infection evokes antibody production and cell-mediated immunity. However, immunity is not total; after reinfection the virus can multiply to a limited degree despite a previous immune response.

Acute ADV infection passes over to a latent infection in which the virus genome persists within the cells of the CNS for a long time. This latent virus infection can be reactivated by stress.

For the diagnosis of AD the clinical symptoms of the herd are more or less conclusive. However, final diagnosis is only possible by means of virus isolation, immunofluorescence tests on tissue sections, or by the determination of antibodies in the serum. Serological tests are also used for detecting infected herds in field surveys and to check the state of sanitation. The neutralisation test is the one most commonly used at present, although the enzyme-linked immunosorbent assay (ELISA) is becoming more and more important. The immunodiffusion test and radioimmunoassay are also used.

Live vaccines and inactivated vaccines are available for protection of pigs against AD. With live vaccines there is a large variation in the degree of attenuation of the modified virus. All modified virus strains multiply in the host and are excreted. Some of them are transmitted to other animals and it cannot be excluded that reversion to virulence occurs during passage. Inactivated vaccines are as efficient as live vaccines, but less hazardous. One difficulty with vaccination with both sorts of vaccines is the blockade of active immunisation by colostrally transmitted maternal antibodies. Vaccination of other species is apparently very ineffective.

Protection of vaccinated pigs against ADV infection is usually not complete and frequently slight clinical symptoms occur. This is due to virus multiplication, which takes place when sufficient amounts of virus have been taken up by the vaccinated animals. The dose of virus required to infect vaccinated pigs is higher than that required for non-immune pigs, but when the infection takes the virus multiplies in the vaccinated animal and invades the CNS. In some cases the virus is also disseminated by leukocytes to other organs and tissues. Furthermore, the infected, vaccinated pigs become latently infected for a long time and thus represent an epizootiological problem.

AD is distributed world wide and is present in most countries of Europe. The incidence of the disease is increasing and areas with dense pig populations are particularly at risk.

From the epizootiological point of view, acutely and chronically infected pigs are the main source of infection and of virus spread. The other species are less important since, in most cases, they die and virus spread is thus interrupted. The most important cause of virus spread over long distances is the trade with persistently infected pigs. Infected boars in cover stations and artificial insemination centres can also disseminate the virus. Rats, cats, dogs and insects seem to be of minor importance for causing virus spread. Air-borne infection over short distances can occur and virus transmission is possible by man, vehicles, food, implements and offals.

Vaccination alone will not lead to eradication. It only reduces or prevents clinical disease. It does not prevent the spread of the virus. Further meausures for the eradication of the virus need to be discussed.

SESSION I

PROPERTIES OF THE VIRUS

Chairman: H. Ludwig

DIFFERENTIATION OF AUJESZKY'S DISEASE VIRUS STRAINS BY RESTRICTION ENDONUCLEASE ANALYSIS OF THE VIRAL DNA'S

A.L.J. Gielkens[1] and A.J.M. Berns[2]

[1] Central Veterinary Institute, Department of Virology, 39, Houtribweg, 8221 RA Lelystad, The Netherlands.

[2] University of Nijmegen, Laboratory of Biochemistry, N21, Geert Grooteplein, 6525 EZ Nijmegen, The Netherlands.

ABSTRACT

Aujeszky's disease virus (ADV) DNA of 16 field isolates, including the four NIA-3 strains with different biological properties, and five modified live virus vaccine strains was analysed by cleavage with restriction endonucleases. After cleavage of the high molecular weight DNA from purified virions or from infected cells, fragments were separated by agarose gel electrophoresis, transferred to nitrocellulose filters and hybridised with radioactive ADV DNA.

The BamH1 and Kpn1 cleavage patterns of virion DNA isolated from the highly virulent isolate NIA-3 could be readily differentiated from that of the vaccine strain MK-25. Digestion of NIA-3 DNA by BamH1 yielded at least 14 fragments with molecular weights between 0.9×10^6 and 26×10^6 daltons. Eight NIA-3 fragments co-migrated with fragments generated by BamH1 cleavage of MK-25 DNA. Cleavage patterns similar to those of virion DNA were obtained when the Southern blotting hybridisation technique was applied to intracellular DNA from NIA-3 or MK-25 infected cells.

The Kpn1 DNA fragment patterns of the five vaccine strains differed markedly from each other and from those of 14 of the field isolates of ADV. These field isolates in turn were also different from each other, although some strains appeared to be more closely related than others. Isolates from two clinical cases of Aujesky's disease (AD) in pigs in the field exhibited DNA fragment patterns identical to those of the modified live virus vaccines used to vaccinate the herd shortly before the problem arose.

These observations suggest that restriction endonuclease analysis of viral DNA may well prove to be an adequate tool for unambiguous identification of ADV isolates from the field.

INTRODUCTION

Aujeszky's disease (AD) is an acute and often fatal nervous condition of domestic and wild animals caused by a herpes virus. The variability in virulence and biological behaviour of field isolates of Aujeszky's disease virus (ADV) raises the question whether virulence and strain-specific markers can be found. The availability of techniques for the detection of such markers would be of practical importance in studies of the epizootiology and in control of the disease;

G. Wittmann, S.A. Hall (eds), Aujeszky's Disease. ISBN-13:978-94-009-7555-2

for example, to distinguish between virulent and vaccine virus strains. In the past, several methods have been described for differentiation of ADV strains based on biological markers. Although some of these methods allowed grouping in virulence classes and sometimes the recognition of a particular vaccine strain, they have not found a wide acceptance.

In the case of herpes simplex virus isolates, intratypic differences have been demonstrated by analysis of virion structural polypeptides and by restriction endonuclease cleavage of virion DNAs (Pereira et al., 1976; Hayward et al., 1975). Comparison of virion, and intracellular polypeptide patterns of virulent and vaccine ADV strains by two dimensional gel electrophoresis yielded no major strain-specific polypeptide markers, although minor differences were observed (unpublished observations). Our second approach involved analysis of field isolates and modified live virus (MLV) vaccines by restriction endonuclease cleavage of virion or intracellular DNAs. In this paper we report on the applicability of this method for identification of ADV isolates.

The ADV genome is a linear, double-stranded DNA molecule of approximately 90×10^6 daltons. It consists of a short unique sequence, bracketed by inverted complementary repeats and a long unique sequence (Ben-Porat et al., 1979). The genomic location of the major DNA fragments generated by the restriction endonucleases *Bam*Hl and *Kpn*l has been described by Rixon and Ben Porat (1979).

MATERIALS AND METHODS

Viruses and cells

Secondary pig kidney cells (PK_2) were grown in Eagle minimal essential medium supplemented with 10% lamb serum and antibiotics at $37^{\circ}C$ in a CO_2 incubator. ADV was propagated by infecting confluent monolayers of PK_2 cells with approximately 1 p.f.u. per cell. The infected cultures were incubated until an extensive cytopathic effect was observed.

The Northern Ireland ADV isolates NIA-1, NIA-2, NIA-3
and NIA-4 were kindly supplied by Dr. J.B. McFerran (Veterinary
Research Laboratories, Belfast, Northern Ireland).

The following modified live virus vaccines were studied:
strains Ercegovac and MK-25 (Tatarov, 1968), produced by
Pharmachim, Sofia, Bulgaria; Duvaxyn, based on Bartha's K strain
(Bartha, 1961) and produced by Duphar B.V., Weesp, the
Netherlands; Ayvac, produced by Pliva, Yugoslavia and Delsuvac,
based on strain BUK TK/650-A (Skoda et al., 1964), produced by
Lab. Dr. de Zeeuw B.V., de Bilt, the Netherlands.

In addition to the above more or less well defined ADV
strains, twelve isolates from the field were studied. Some of
these isolates were obtained from diseased pigs that had been
vaccinated a few days previously.

Extraction and purification of DNA

For the preparation of NIA-3 and MK-25 DNA, virus was
purified from the medium of infected BHK-suspension cell cultures. The partially purified virus was lysed in 50 mM Tris-
hydrochloride (pH 7.8), 10 mM EDTA and 0.5% sodium dodecyl-
sulfate (SDS) at room temperature. After addition of proteinase
K (100 µg/ml final concentration, Boehringer) the lysate was
incubated at 37°C for 1 h. The extracted viral DNA was then
purified by two cycles of equilibrium NaI buoyant density
centrifugation as described by Walboomers and ter Schegget (1976).

For the isolation of intracellular DNA, cells were
harvested between 15 and 20 h after infection. Cells were
pelleted by centrifugation and resuspended in TNE (50 mM Tris-
hydrochloride (pH 7.8), 0.15 M NaCl, 10 mM/EDTA) buffer.
Proteinase K was added to a final concentration of 100 µg/ml
and the cells were lysed by addition of SDS to a final concentration of 1%. The lysate was incubated at 37°C for 2 h.
Subsequently, the solution was extracted twice or three times
with buffer-saturated phenol- m-cresol, twice with chloroform-
isoamylalcohol (25 : 1) and the nucleic acids were precipitated
with two volumes of ethanol. The precipitate was dissolved in
TE (10 mM Tris-hydrochloride (pH 7.5), 1 mM EDTA) buffer and
digested with 20 µg/ml of RNase A (Boehringer) for 60 min at

room temperature. This was followed by digestion with proteinase K for 60 min at 37°C. The digest was extracted once with
chloroform-phenol (1 : 1), once with chloroform-isoamylalcohol
(25 : 1) and the DNA was precipitated with ethanol.

Restriction endonuclease analysis

Viral and intracellular DNA was cleaved with the
restriction endonucleases *Bam*H1 and *Kpn*1 as described by van der
Putten et al. (1979). The digested DNA was fractionated on
0.6% agarose gels in a buffer containing 40 mM Tris base, 1 mM
EDTA, and 5 mM sodium acetate, adjusted with acetic acid to pH
7.9. DNA fragments were identified either by ethidium bromide
staining or by the Southern blotting hybridisation technique
(Southern, 1975), using NIA-3 DNA labelled with ^{32}P by the nick
translation procedure (Berns et al., 1980).

RESULTS

Restriction endonuclease digestion of NIA-3 and MK-25 DNA

The cleavage patterns of the viral DNAs of the highly
virulent NIA-3 strain and the vaccine strain MK-25 with either
*Bam*H1 or *Kpn*1 are shown in Figure 1. The digestion products
ranged in molecular weight from 0.9 x 10^6 to 26 x 10^6 daltons.
Comparison of the cleavage patterns revealed that both enzymes
clearly discriminated between NIA-3 and MK-25. Cleavage of
NIA-3 DNA with *Bam*H1 yielded at least 14 DNA fragments of which
8 co-migrated with fragment bands generated by *Bam*H1 digestion
of MK-25 DNA. *Kpn*1 digestion of NIA-3 DNA resulted in at least
12 DNA fragments, of which several were co-migrating with *Kpn*1
fragment bands of MK-25. Mapping of the *Bam*H1 and *Kpn*1 restriction endonuclease cleavage sites of NIA-3 and MK-25 DNA will
be required to prove that co-migrating fragments are indeed
derived from common regions of the genome of both isolates.

All fragment bands in digests of purified NIA-3 and MK-25
DNA detected by ethidium bromide staining of the gels were also
detected with ^{32}P-labelled NIA-3 DNA as hybridisation probe.
This observation indicates a high degree of genetic relatedness
between the NIA-3 and MK-25 isolates. Therefore, we believe

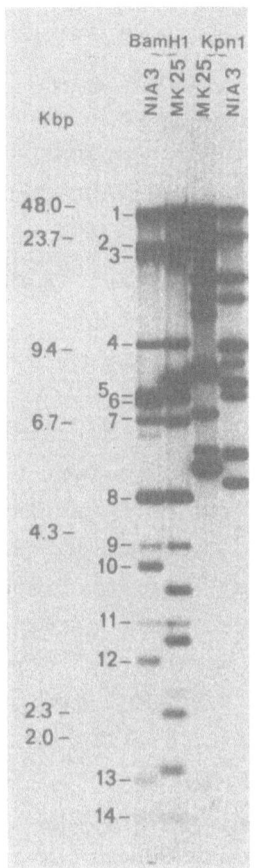

Fig. 1.   Fig. 2.

Fig. 1.   Autoradiographs of restriction endonuclease digested ADV-DNAs.
Virion DNA of the highly virulent strain NIA-3 and the MLV vaccine
strain MK-25 were cleaved with BamHl and Kpnl. The DNA fragments
were separated by electrophoresis in O.6% agarose gels and transferred to nitrocellulose filters. ^{32}P-labelled NIA-3 DNA was
hybridised to the filters and the viral fragment bands were visual-
ised by autoradiography. Designations of NIA-3 BamHl fragments are
indicated next to the corresponding fragment profile. Standard
molecular weight markers were run in the same gel i.e. a mixture
of lambda DNA and lambda DNA cleaved with HindIII.

Fig. 2.   Autoradiographs of Kpnl cleavage patterns of virion or intracellular DNA from virulent and MLV vaccine ADV strains. Slots
1 - 5, intracellular DNA from the vaccines Ercegovac, MK-25,
Duvaxyn, Ayvac and Delsuvac, respectively; 6 and 7 van Doorn and
NIA-3 intracellular DNA, respectively; 8 and 9 NIA-3 and MK-25
virion DNA, respectively. Designations of NIA-3 Kpnl fragments
are indicated at the right. Analysis performed as described in
Fig. 1.

that ^{32}P-labelled DNA is an adequate probe for comparative studies of ADV strains by the Southern blotting hybridisation technique.

No differences were observed between the digestion patterns of DNA isolated from cells infected with NIA-3 or MK-25 and their viral DNAs (Figure 2, lanes 7,8 and 2,9). For this reason, all further analyses were performed with intracellular DNA from ADV infected cells.

Differences among vaccine strains

*Kpn*I digestion of five modified live virus (MLV) vaccine strains yielded a characteristic and reproducible pattern of electrophoretically separable DNA fragments for each vaccine strain (Figure 2). DNA fragment bands A, B, C, J and L were co-migrating among all vaccine virus strains. The *Kpn*I fragment D was present in all isolates, except Delsuvac. The sizes of certain other fragments showed considerable variation. For example, many differences were found in the E/F and I region. Thus, the *Kpn*I restriction fragment patterns of the DNAs allowed identification of each MLV vaccine.

The vaccine virus strains studied were also readily differentiated from the Dutch isolate van Doorn, which is of moderate virulence (Figure 2, lane 6), and the highly virulent strain NIA-3 (Figure 2, lane 7).

The electrophoretic profiles of the *Kpn*I digests of the MLV vaccines Ercegovac, Duvaxyn, Ayvac and Delsuvac, contained a variable number of minor bands, occurring in sub-molar quantities. Since the vaccines studied were not plaque purified, occurrence of minor bands may be accounted for by defective genomes or mixtures of closely related strains in these vaccine stocks. Results of recent experiments demonstrated minor differences between the electrophoretic profiles of vaccine stocks and plaque purified vaccine strains.

Differences between field isolates of ADV

The genomes of field isolates of clinical cases of AD were examined. Some isolates were derived from pigs vaccinated with inactivated or MLV vaccines against AD shortly before clinical signs of the disease appeared. Isolate 10 is a rabbit passage of isolate 9.

The *Kpn*l digestion patterns of ADV isolates 1 and 3 were indistinguishable from those of plaque purified isolates of the MLV vaccines Ercegovac and MK-25, respectively (Figure 3). These isolates were also identified with the restriction endonuclease *Bam*Hl (not shown). The remaining isolates exhibited DNA fragment patterns different from those of the MLV vaccines studied.

Comparison of the *Kpn*l cleavage patterns of the ADV isolates 2, 4, 5, 6, 7, 8, 9 and 11 shows that all isolates were different (Figure 3). Some virus isolates had very similar DNA fragment patterns (compare 2 and 8, 5 and 7, Figure 3) which differed by only one band, others showed much less matching of fragments. NIA-3 shared DNA fragments A, B, C, J and L with all other isolates, suggesting that these fragments represent constant regions of the ADV genome. No differences in the *Kpn*l restriction endonuclease fragment patterns were observed between isolates 9 and 10, the latter was obtained after passage of isolate 9 in a rabbit.

Differences among isolates with specific biological properties

In Northern Ireland four ADV strains have been isolated and characterised as regards their biological properties (McFerran and Dow, 1965; Baskerville, 1972; Baskerville et al., 1973). Virus strain NIA-1 is a virulent neurotropic isolate. Strain NIA-2 is a virulent isolate causing striking lung lesions and sever rhinitis. Experimentally, NIA-1 and NIA-2 cause 5 - 20% mortality in 7-week-old pigs. Strain NIA-3 is a highly virulent isolate causing 80 - 100% deaths in 7-week-old pigs. The fourth strain, NIA-4, isolated from a cow suspected of malignant catarrhal fever, was found to be non-pathogenic at least for the animal species tested (Baskerville et al., 1973).

Since it may be expected that differences in biological properties reflect nucleotide sequence differences within the ADV genome, the Northern Ireland strains were analysed by restriction endonuclease digestion. Cleavage of intracellular

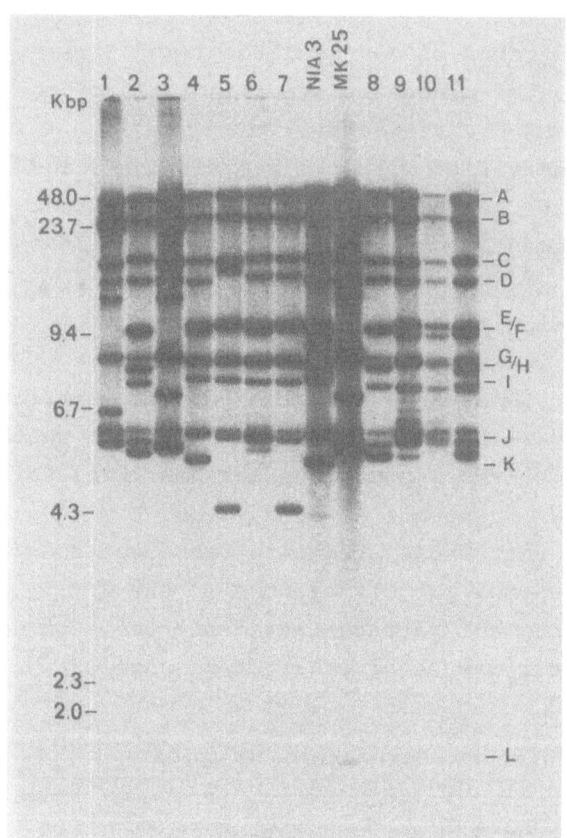 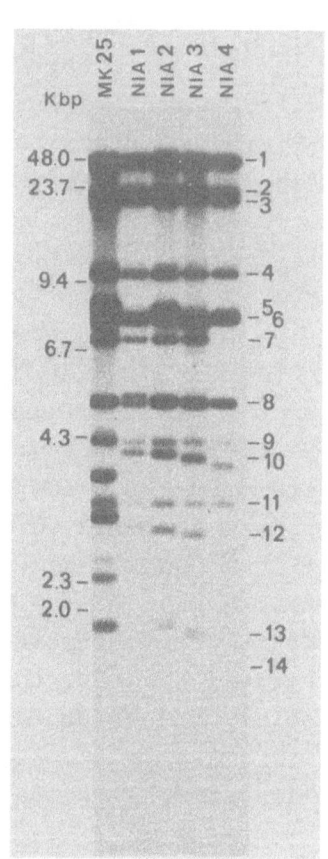

Fig. 3   Fig. 4

Fig. 3   Autoradiographs of *Kpn*1 cleavage patterns of intracellular DNA from
         field isolates of ADV. Numbered tracks correspond to different
         field isolates, except number 10 which was isolated from a rabbit
         infected with isolate 9. Designations of NIA-3 *Kpn*1 fragments are
         indicated at the right. Analysis performed as described in Fig. 1.

Fig. 4   Autoradiographs of *Bam*H1 cleavage patterns of ADV strains with dif-
         ferent biological properties. Designations of NIA-3 *Bam*H1 fragments
         are indicated at the right. Analysis performed as described in Fig. 1.

DNA of each isolate by *Bam*Hl generated a characteristic DNA fragment pattern distinguishable from the other strains (Figure 4). Comparison of the patterns showed co-migration of eight fragment bands (1, 2, 3, 4, 8, 9, 11 and 14, Figure 4) among all strains. Whether one of the fragment bands numbered 5 and 6 were co-migrating among these strains is uncertain, due to the limited resolution of these bands. A striking difference between NIA-4 and the other strains is the absence in the former isolate of a DNA band corresponding in size to fragment 7. Possibly, nucleotide sequences of the NIA-4 genome corresponding to this region are at least partly deleted. Further studies are needed to clarify the significance of this finding.

DISCUSSION

Virion and intracellular DNAs of field isolate of ADV and of MLV vaccines were cleaved in fragments with the restriction endonucleases *Bam*Hl or *Kpn*l. The DNA fragments generated were separated by agarose gel electrophoresis and identified by Southern blotting hybridisations with ^{32}P-labelled NIA-3 DNA. When the *Kpn*l digested virion DNA of the MLV vaccine MK-25 was analysed with this technique, a DNA fragment pattern was obtained identical to the electrophoretic profile of *Kpn*l cleaved MK-25 DNA in ethidium bromide stained gels. Thus, although the *Bam*Hl and *Kpn*l restriction endonuclease fragment patterns of NIA-3 and MK-25 l NA differed significantly, all DNA fragments of MK-25 were recognised with the ^{32}P-labelled NIA-3 probe. Therefore, the ^{32}P-labelled NIA-3 DNA is an adequate probe for identification of different ADV isolates.

The intracellular DNAs of several ADV isolates from clinical cases were examined. The variation in the DNA fragment patterns generated by *Kpn*l was sufficient to distinguish among these isolates. For a few isolates rather similar DNA fragment patterns were obtained, whereas others showed considerable variation. Two isolates from pigs that had been vaccinated 5 - 14 days before clinical signs of AD appeared, showed DNA fragment patterns identical to the commercially available MLV vaccines MK-25 and Ercegovac, respectively. A number of the

isolates obtained under similar conditions gave a clearly
different pattern from the MLV vaccine used in the field.

Comparable results were obtained when the intracellular
DNAs of five commercially available MLV vaccines were analysed
by cleavage with *Kpn*1. Each vaccine exhibited a characteristic
DNA fragment pattern, that differed from the other vaccines
examined. Some minor, presumably submolar, bands were present
in the cleavage patterns of all vaccine strains, except MK-25.
Although, definite proof awaits further work, these minor bands
could be due to defective virus or closely related ADV variants
in the vaccine stocks used for infection of the cells. This is
supported by recent results from restriction endonuclease
analysis of plaque purified vaccine strains.

Since it may be anticipated that specific sequences
within the ADV genome are related with biological functions of
the virus, we examined four ADV strains known to possess different biological properties. Analysis of the intracellular
DNA of the Northern Ireland strains NIA-1, NIA-2, NIA-3 and
NIA-4 by *Bam*H1 cleavage indicated differences in the genome
organisation of these strains. Several DNA fragments, e.g. 5,
6, 10, 12 and 13, show considerable variation in size among the
NIA strains. This size variation could be due to insertions or
deletions in the respective fragments. In addition, fragment
band 7, which is present in all virulent isolates, is missing
in the DNA digest of avirulent NIA-4 virus. Possibly, this
could point to an unusual deletion of nucleotide sequences in
this region of the NIA-4 genome. Co-migration of the fragment
bands 1, 2, 3, 4, 9, 11 and 14 suggests that these fragments
are identical or closely related and thus may originate from
more conservative parts of the ADV genome.

The results of this study show that application of
restriction endonuclease analysis provides a valuable tool for
the identification of ADV field isolates. In addition, the
possibility to distinguish and characterise ADV isolates will
be beneficial in studies on pathogenesis, epizootiology and
control of the disease.

REFERENCES

Bartha, A. 1961. Experimental reduction of virulence of Aujeszky's disease
    virus. Magy. Allatorv. Lap. 16, 42-45.
Baskerville, A. 1972. Ultrastructural changes in the pulmonary airways of
    pigs infected with a strain of Aujeszky's disease virus. Res. Vet. Sci.,
    13, 127-132.
Baskerville, A., McFerran, J.B. and Dow, C. 1973. Aujeszky's disease in
    pigs. Vet. Bull. 43, 465-480.
Ben-Porat, T., Rixon, F.J. and Blakenship, M. 1979. Analysis of the struc-
    ture of the genome of pseudorabies virus. Virology, 95, 285-294.
Berns, A.J.M., Lai, M.H.T., Bosselman, R.A., McKennett, M.A., Bacheler, L.T.,
    Fan, H., Robanus Maandag, E.C., v.d. Putten, H. and Verma, I.H. 1980.
    Molecular cloning of unintegrated and a portion of integrated Moloney
    murine leukemia viral DNA in bacteriophage lambda. J. Virol., 36,
    254-263.
Hayward, G.S., Frenkel, N. and Roizman, B. 1975. Anatomy of herpes simplex
    virus DNA: strain differneces and heterogeneity in the locations of
    restriction endonuclease cleavage sites. Proc. Nat. Acad. Sci. USA, 72,
    1768-1772.
McFerran, J.B. and Dow, C. 1965. The distribution of the virus of Aujeszky's
    disease (pseudorabies virus) in experimentally infected swine. Am. J.
    Vet. Res. 26, 631-635.
Pereira, L., Cassai, E. Honess, R.W., Roizman, B., Termi, M. and Nahmias,
    A.J. 1976. Variability in the structural polypeptides of herpes simplex
    virus 1 strains: potential application in molecular epidemiology. Infec.
    Immun., 13, 211-220.
Rixon, F.J. and Ben-Porat, T. 1979. Structural evolution of the DNA of pseu-
    dorabies-defective viral particles. Virology, 97, 151-163.
Skoda, R., Braumer, I., Sadecky, E. and Mayer, V. 1964. Immunization against
    Aujeszky's disease with live vaccine. I. Attenuation of virus and some
    properties of attenuated strains. Acta Virol., Prague, 8, 1-9.
Southern, W.M. 1975. Detection of specific sequences among DNA fragments se-
    parated by gel electrophoresis. J. Mol. Biol., 98, 503-517.
Tatarov, G. 1968. Apathogener mutant des Aujeszky-virus, induziert von 5-
    Jodo-2-Deoxyuridin (JUDR). Zentbl. Vet. Med., 15B, 847-853.
Van der Putten, H., Terwindt, E., Berns, A. and Jaenisch, R. 1979. The in-
    tegration sites of endogenous and exogenous Moloney murine leukemia
    virus. Cell, 18, 109-116.
Walboomers, J.M.M. and ter Schegget, J. 1976. A new method for the isolation
    of herpes simplex virus type 2 DNA. Virology, 74, 256-258.

THE GENOMES OF DIFFERENT FIELD ISOLATES OF AUJESZKY'S DISEASE VIRUS

H. Ludwig, B. Heppner and S. Herrmann

Institut für Virologie, Freie Universität Berlin,
Nordufer 20 (im Robert Koch-Institut), 1000 Berlin 65,
Federal Republic of Germany.

ABSTRACT

A variety of Aujeszky's disease virus (ADV) isolates have been differentiated by molecular biological techniques. Restriction enzyme analysis of the purified DNAs with Kpn I, Hind III, Hpa I, Bam H I, and Sal I allowed an easy and clear separation of the genomes. As based on the DNA patterns four major classes of ADV strains could be constructed. Their epizootological importance is under further investigation.

INTRODUCTION

ADV strains have not been confidently differentiated by biological techniques and are considered to represent one serotype although a variety of biological markers are known (Bartha et al., 1969; Kaplan, 1969; Lloyd and Baskerville, 1978; Toma et al., 1979). A correlation of the function of virion components with genome structure as the basis for better understanding of virulence in Aujeszky's disease (AD) is not yet possible and is just being investigated in other herpesvirus systems. The application of the 'molecular fingerprinting' technique to micro- and macroepidemiological studies of herpesvirus infections has shown that this will be an appropriate tool to trace origin and spread of strains (Buchman et al., 1979; Engels et al., 1981). As shown in this report which extends earlier data (Heppner et al., 1981) a successful differentiation of ADV strains can be accomplished using restriction endonuclease fingerprinting of viral DNAs.

MATERIALS AND METHODS

ADV strains originating from different parts of Germany, from other virological laboratories in Europe or from fatal cases in dogs and cats in Berlin are listed in Table 1. All these strains seemed to be involved in the death of those animals. Virus growth conditions and some details on DNA

G. Wittmann, S.A. Hall (eds), Aujeszky's Disease. ISBN-13:978-94-009-7555-2

TABLE 1

TITRATION AND PRELIMINARY GROUPING[1] OF ADV ISOLATES

Code	Origin	Titre KID_{50}	Typing after digestion with restriction enzymes:				
			Kpn I	Hind III	Hpa I	Bam H I	Sal I
DEK	refer.	$10^{-4.6}$	I	I	I	I	II
JP	pig	$10^{-4.3}$		I	II		
A48	pig	$10^{-5.3}$		I	II		
VO/12/9	pig	$10^{-2.67}$	I	I	I	I	I
VO/12/42	pig	$10^{-4.67}$	I	I	I	I	I
VO/12/46	pig	$10^{-3.67}$	I	I	I	I	I
V9/12/1	pig	10^{-4}		I	I		
VO/1/3	pig	10^{-4}		I	I		
VO/3/2	pig	$10^{-3.81}$		I	I		
VO/3/4	dog	$10^{-4.5}$			I		
VO/4/4	dog	$10^{-3.81}$		I	I		
VO/5/2	dog	$10^{-4.57}$		I	I		
VO/8/49	dog	$10^{-3.38}$		I	I		
VO/8/53	dog	10^{-3}		I	II		
VO/4/2	cat	$10^{-5.23}$	I	I	III	II	II
VO/4/2pp2	cat	$10^{-4.57}$	I	I	III	II	II
VO/9/3	cat	$10^{-4.3}$	I	I	I	I	I
VO/9/4	cat	$10^{-2.5}$	I	I	III	II	II
VO/12/39	cat	$10^{-4.5}$	I	I	I	I	III
VO/12/41	cat	$10^{-4.67}$	I	I	I	I	I
VO/9/2	cattle	$10^{-4.67}$	I	II	I	III	II
VO/12/5	fox	$10^{-3.67}$	I	I	I	I	I
VO/12/13	bear	10^{-3}	II	I	I	I	III

1) Grouping was done according to the frequency of appearance of the same
   DNA pattern in all isolates obtained after digestion with each restriction enzyme. No I stands for the group assembling most of the strains
   with identical patterns; compare also Figures 2 and 3.

analysis can be found in earlier papers (Ludwig et al., 1972; Ludwig et al., 1974). For analysis of the DNA 10^9 to 10^{10} virus particles were purified, lysed with SDS, digested with protein- ase K, followed by extraction with phenol and chloroform/isoamyl- alcohol and precipitation of the DNA with ethanol. Restriction enzyme digestion and subsequent analysis of the DNA fragments in agarose gels followed essentially standard procedures (Nathans and Smith, 1975).

RESULTS AND CONCLUSIONS

ADV DNAs of different strains which have a buoyant density of 1.731 g/ml in CsCl cannot be separated by analytical ultracentrifugation or by equilibrium density centrifugation in CsCl of doubly labelled (^{3}H-thymidine and ^{14}C-thymidine) DNAs (Ludwig, 1972; Heppner et al., unpublished).

The ADV genome has a characteristic structure resembling that of IBR/IPV virus with repetitive DNA sequences at one end of the molecule, which is different from HSV and BHM virus DNAs (Figure 1). Restriction enzyme analysis of the genomes of 22 independent ADV isolates and a reference strain revealed the results summarised in Table 1.

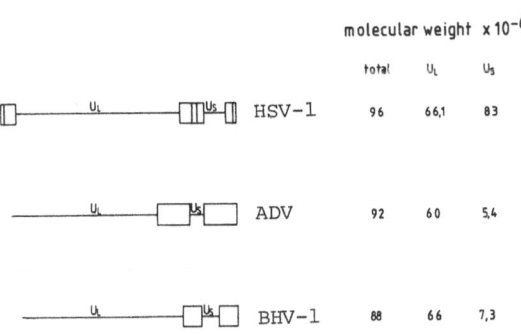

Fig. 1. Sequence arrangements of the ADV genome in comparison to those of BHV-1 (IBR/IPV virus) or HSV-1 and BHV-2 (BHM virus; not shown) redrawn from Buchman and Roizman (1978); Skare, J. (personal communication).

18

Kpn I and Hind III cleaved the DNAs into 11 or 12 and 3 or 4 fragments, respectively (Figures 2 and 3) (Ben-Porat and Rixon, 1979). From these 2 types of DNA patterns the majority fell into group I (Table 1)

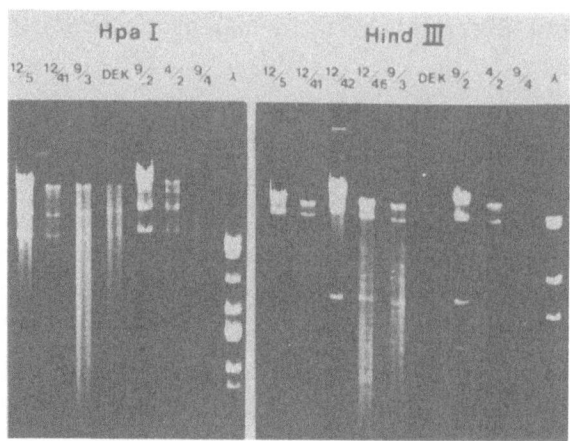

Fig. 2. Patterns of Hpa I and Hind III digests of ADV-DNA; 0.6% agarose slab gels, 35 V, 24 h.

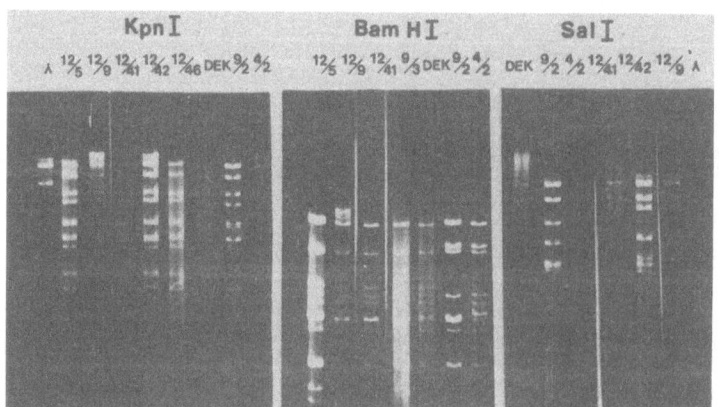

Fig. 3. Patterns of Kpn I, Bam H I, Sal I digests of ADV-DNA; 0.7% agarose slab gels, 35 V, 18 h.

The enzyme Hpa I cleaved the DNAs in 3 to 5 fragments, whereas with Bam H I and Sal I a considerably higher number of fragments was generated (Figures 2 and 3). With each enzyme 3 types of DNA patterns were obvious. Sal I seems to allow further differentiation of strains (Lomniczi, personal communication).

A comparison of the DNA patterns made it possible to group ADV isolates into classes A to D. On the basis of our data the majority of the strains seem to be completely identical whereas others shared varying degrees of common cleavage sites on their DNAs (Figure 4, Table 1).

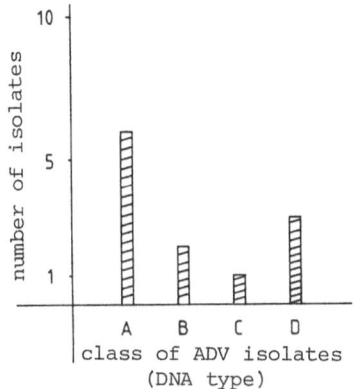

Fig. 4.   Class A represents isolates which belong to the most frequently appearing group. They were all identical when the DNAs were digested with 5 enzymes. Class B: identical in 4; class C: in 3; class D: in 2 DNA patterns with class A after restriction enzyme analysis with the 5 enzymes given in Table 1.

Although a limited number of ADV strains has been tested it can be assumed that class A virus is most widespread in the animal population, since it could be found in almost every group of fatally diseased animals. It is furthermore surprising that a high degree of similarity in DNA patterns of ADV isolates exists, which emphasises the genome stability of this herpes-virus under field conditions. Investigations are underway to use this kind of DNA analysis for epizootological studies. Additionally some of the strains might serve as an appropriate tool to dissect genome parts involved in important biological functions of ADV.

20

REFERENCES

Bartha, A., Belak, S. and Benyeda, J., 1969. Trypsin- and heat-resistance of some strains of the herpesvirus group. Acta Vet. Acad. Sci. Hung., 19, 97-99.

Ben-Porat, T. and Rixon, F.J., 1979. Replication of herpesvirus DNA; IV. Analysis of concatemers. Virology, 94, 61-70.

Buchman, T.G. and Roizman, B., 1978. Anatomy of bovine mammillitis DNA. II. Size and arrangements of the deoxynucleotide sequences. J. Virol., 27, 239-254.

Buchman, T.G., Roizman, B. and Nahmias, A.J., 1979. Demonstration of exogenous genital reinfection with herpes simplex virus type 2 by restriction endonuclease fingerprinting of viral DNA. J. Infect. Dis., 140, 295-304.

Engels, M., Steck, F. and Wyler, R., 1981. Comparison of the genomes of IBR and IPV virus strains by means of restriction enzyme analysis. Arch. Virol., 67, 169-174.

Heppner, B., Darai, G., Podesta, B., Pauli, G. and Ludwig, H., 1981. Strain differences in pseudorabies viruses. Med. Microbiol. Immunol., 169, 128.

Kaplan, A.S., 1969. Herpes simplex and pseudorabies viruses. Virol. Monographs, 5 (Springer, Berlin).

Lloyd, G. and Baskerville, A., 1978. *In vitro* markers to differentiate an avirulent from a virulent strain of Aujeszky's disease virus. Vet. Microbiol., 3, 65-70.

Ludwig, H., Biswal, N. and Benyesh-Melnick, M., 1972. Studies on the relatedness of herpesviruses through DNA-DNA hybridization. Virology, 49, 95-101.

Ludwig, H., 1972. Untersuchungen am genetischen Material von Herpesviren. Med. Microbiol. Immunol., 157, 186-238.

Ludwig, H., Becht, H. and Rott, R., 1974. Inhibition of herpesvirus-induced cell fusion by Concanavalin A, antisera, and 2 deoxy-D-glucose. J. Virol., 14, 307-314.

Nathans, D. and Smith, H.O., 1975. Restriction endonucleases in the analysis and restructuring of DNA molecules. Ann. Rev. Biochem., 44, 273-293.

Toma, B., Brun, A., Chappuis, G. and Terre, J., 1979. Propriétés biologiques d'une souche thermosensible (Alfort 26) de virus de la maladie d'Aujeszky. Rec. Méd. Vét., 155, 245-252.

GENERAL DISCUSSION

H. Ludwig (Federal Republic of Germany) Dr. Gielkens, in all
cases you used labelled DNA from one strain; how are you able
to detect fragments which might be different from that one
strain?

A.L.J. Gielkens (Netherlands) At present, for differentiation,
it can be used of course. As we purify more strains, MK25 and
so on, and then use normal techniques with ethidium bromide
colouring we find the patterns of those strains and the labelled
patterns are identical. But of course, for example, for NIA-4,
you are missing band no.7. You have to make a probe from it to
be sure. But I have the impression that the genetic information is strongly related. Of course, there are differences
with restriction enzymes but they are so closely related that
you can use such a probe to differentiate the whole strains.

H. Ludwig Yes, but I think it is a little more laborious.

A.L.J. Gielkens Yes. My impression is that all strains are
different although sometimes there are only very minor differences.

H.-J. Rziha (Federal Republic of Germany) What multiplicity of
infection have you found in the cells?

A.L.J. Gielkens Very low multiplicity, about one.

H.-J. Rziha How can you exclude the formation of defective
DNA? You have some small fragments; it may be that if you
have defective DNA this formation is very readily achieved
after infection with ADV. So you have the reiteration of some
and you get a new small fragment and the loss of the large one.
Can you exclude this formation?

A.L.J. Gielkens During the experiment, when we infect cells
and then collect these cells after 15 hours, that we have
defective particles formed during that time? I don't believe
this is so. I should also say that we have cloned all strains
and the patterns are identical.

H. Ludwig   In one or two passages from tissue culture you
have already had differences in the pattern. This surprised
me.

A.L.J. Gielkens   When you have a strain which is not homo-
geneous, and when you have a field isolate, it is quite possible
that you have two viruses present. The cloning was done afterwards; when you clone it you see a difference.

H. Ludwig   Our experience was that if you use the original
population and cut it, you might have some differences through
the different clones. However, following up different clones,
they are absolutely identical. I think that agrees with our
understanding of the herpes DNA - it will not mutate or reassort
quickly.

A.L.J. Gielkens   That's right. This is also known for the
herpes simplex virus; there are many strains but they are
stable.

O.C. Straub (Federal Republic of Germany)   Dr. Gielkens, have you
ever checked early and late isolates from the same outbreak,
or early and late isolates from the same animal?

A.L.J. Gielkens   Not yet. We have only had these isolates in
the laboratory. We are hoping now to look more closely in the
field and to compare such isolates although I do have one
latently infected animal which yielded the same virus after
corticosteroid treatment.

H. Ludwig   I think one of our Hungarian colleagues, Lomniza,
will solve that problem because he is doing similar studies at
the moment - micro epizootiology - several isolates from one
pig. It appears that they will not easily change in their
pattern.

ANTIGENIC COMPONENTS OF AUJESZKY'S DISEASE VIRUS

G. Pauli, K. Bund and B. Podesta

Institut für Virologie
Freie Universität Berlin
Nordufer 20 (im Robert Koch-Institut), 1000 Berlin 65
Federal Republic of Germany.

ABSTRACT

Aujeszky's disease virus (ADV) strains or isolates from field cases could not be distinguished by serological methods. In ADV infected cells up to 10 different proteins ranging in molecular weights from 40 000 – 200 000 could be detected by immunoprecipitation tests and SDS PAGE analysis. Six of the proteins were glycosylated. Individual antisera prepared against precipitation bands obtained by immunoelectrophoresis gave rise to antibodies neutralising ADV. One of the sera with high neutralising potency recognised only one glycoprotein which had an apparent molecular weight of 80 000.

INTRODUCTION

Herpesviruses have a complex structure which makes it difficult to analyse and characterise virus subunits and limits our knowledge about the functional importance of viral components during infection. Virus proteins involved in the immune defence of the infected host are of major interest. In ADV infections, which are of great economic importance, little is known about the major immunogenic proteins and antigens. In this report preliminary experiments on serological and biochemical properties of ADV specific proteins will be given.

MATERIALS AND METHODS

Virus

The DEK strain and field isolates from cats and dogs were used (Ludwig et al., this publication). Virus was propagated in primary rabbit kidney cell cultures (Pauli and Ludwig, 1977). For immunisation purposes cell cultures were washed 5 x with medium containing rabbit serum and supplemented for 5 days with medium (2% rabbit serum) prior to infection.

G. Wittmann, S.A. Hall (eds), Aujeszky's Disease. ISBN-13:978-94-009-7555-2

Immune sera

Sera directed against ADV proteins were obtained by immunising rabbits 3 x with detergent lysed ADV infected cells (approx. 5×10^7 cells) in Freund's adjuvant. These sera showed high neutralising antibody titres. Antisera directed against distinct immunoprecipitates were prepared according to Vestergaard (1975).

Neutralisation of ADV

This was performed with the plaque reduction test essentially as detailed by Pauli and Ludwig (1977).

Antigen preparation

Lysates were made from infected cells by treatment with Triton-x 100 (Norrild et al., 1978) or with Nonidet NP-40 and deoxycholate (Pauli and Ludwig, 1977). Crossed immunoelectrophoresis followed procedures outlined by Axelsen et al. (1975). The analysis of precipitates on SDS polyacrylamide gels obtained either by immunoelectrophoresis or by the indirect immunoprecipitation technique was carried out as described elsewhere (Pauli and Ludwig, 1977).

Labelling of ADV infected cells

Cell monolayers were infected with a m.o.i. of 10. Five hours post infection the growth medium was replaced by labelling medium containing radioactive precursors for protein or glycoprotein synthesis (Pauli and Ludwig, 1977).

RESULTS

Indirect immunoprecipitation tests revealed that up to 10 proteins, ranging in apparent molecular weights between 40 000 to 200 000 were recognised by convalescent sera from pigs or by hyperimmune sera from pigs or rabbits. Six of these proteins were glycosylated (Figure 1). With a different technique, the crossed immunoelectrophoresis, up to 10 precipitation arcs could be demonstrated (Figure 2). Neither method allowed discrimination of ADV strains or isolates from field cases.

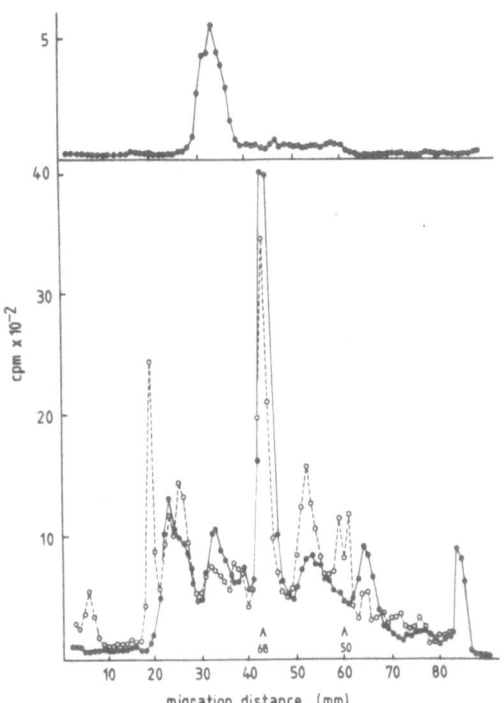

Fig. 1. Analysis of precipitates on polyacrylamide gels. Lower part:
o---o ^{3}H-amino acids labelled ADV proteins and ●——● ^{3}H-glucosamine
labelled glycoproteins precipitated with a convalescent pig serum.
Upper part: Analysis of a precipitate obtained with antiserum
prepared against band 3 (see Figure 2) using ^{3}H-glucosamine
labelled infected cell antigens. The samples were analysed on
parallel gels (8%). For details see Pauli and Ludwig (1977).

In an approach to distinguish field isolates, cross
neutralisation experiments were performed using four strains
and the corresponding polyvalent antisera. No significant
differences could be obtained in this test (data not shown).

In attempts to study the antigenic structures that could
be involved in the immune defence reaction, monoprecipitin
sera directed against four single immunoprecipitation arcs were

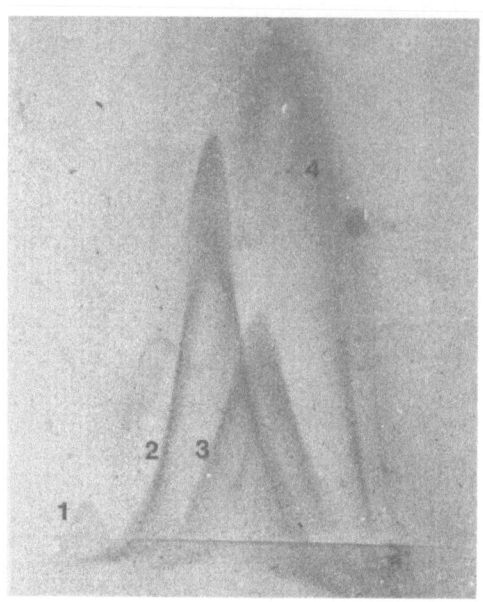

Fig. 2. Crossed immunoelectrophoresis in agarose gels. ADV cellular
         antigens were subjected to first dimension electrophoresis
         followed by second dimension electrophoresis into ADV specific
         polyvalent antibodies (15 µl/cm^2). Further details of the tech-
         nique have been reported (Norrild et al., 1978).

tested for the capacity to inactivate ADV. Three out of the
four precipitation bands induced neutralising antibodies
(Figure 3). The analysis of the antisera by the indirect
immunoprecipitation technique revealed that all sera except one
precipitated more than one glycoprotein. This result showed
that the antigens recognised in immunoelectrophoresis were of
more or less complexity. Our data are in agreement with
results obtained in another system (Norrild et al., 1978).
The antiserum prepared against band 3 precipitated only one
glycoprotein with an apparent molecular weight of 80 000
(Figure 1). Comparable results were obtained when the individual
precipitation arcs were analysed on SDS polyacrylamide gels.

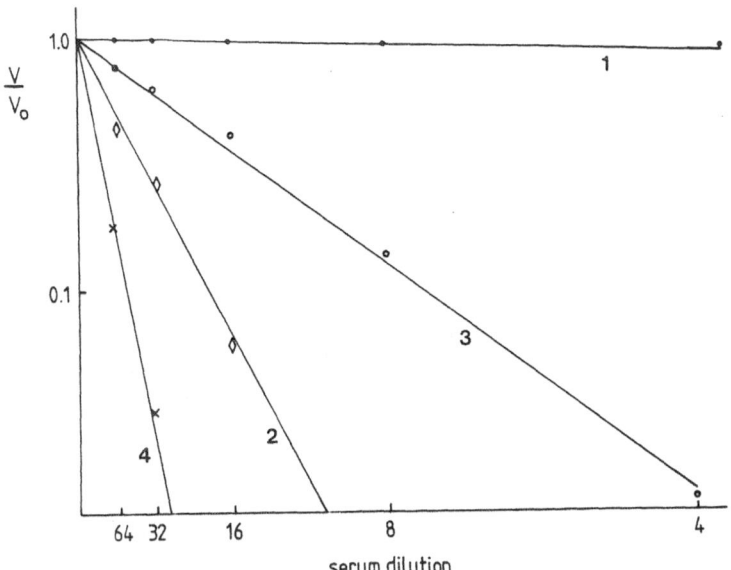

Fig. 3. Neutralisation of ADV. Four individual sera prepared against agarose precipitates (see Figure 2) were tested in a plaque reduction test. V/V_0 is the fractional reduction in plaque counts at the given serum dilution.

In conclusion it could be shown that at least one major immunogenic component, a glycoprotein with an apparent molecular weight of 80 000 could be identified. Further analyses of the role of other glycoproteins which could also induce neutralising antibodies are under investigation at present.

REFERENCES

Axelsen, N.H., Krøll, J. and Weeke, B., 1975. A manual of quantitative immunoelectrophoresis. (Universitetsforlaget, Oslo, Bergen, Tromsø).

Norrild, B., Ludwig, H. and Rott., R., 1978. Identification of a common antigen of herpes simplex virus, bovine herpes mammillitis virus and B virus. J. Virol., 26, 712-717.

Pauli, G. and Ludwig, H., 1977. Immunoprecipitation of herpes simplex virus type 1 antigens with different antisera and human cerebrospinal fluids. Arch. Virol., 53, 139-155.

Vestergaard, B.F., 1975. Production of antiserum against a specific herpes simplex type 2 antigen. Scand. J. Immunology 4, Suppl. 2, 203-206.

DISCUSSION

<u>V. Moennig</u> *(Federal Republic of Germany)* I have a general question
to those people who work on differentiation of the virus strains.
Have you already established that monoclonal antibodies are of
use for differentiation of different strains of Aujeszky's virus
or, if not, do you think it would be useful to do this?

<u>G. Pauli</u> *(Federal Republic of Germany)* I think it would be useful
but first we must know which proteins are really involved. I
think the method of DNA fingerprinting is much easier than using
monoclonal antibodies to differentiate the strains. However,
I do think it is very important to know which structures of the
virus are really involved in the defence of the organism against
an infection. It may be that then one could immunise with
really pure proteins.

<u>A.L.J. Gielkens</u> *(Netherlands)* With monoclonal antibodies, you
have to make one against each virus strain you have isolated
because you detect only one determinant. You see one virus and
you don't see the other ones. When you use DNA cleavage and
fragment analysis you always see a virus and you can recognise
a particular pattern, a particular strain. This is not
possible if you use monoclonal antibodies.

<u>H. Ludwig</u> *(Federal Republic of Germany)* I think it would be very
fortunate if you had that monoclonal antibody covering the
neutralising site, because I think everyone still agrees that
Aujeszky's disease virus is one serotype, so we might believe
that it neutralises only one major antigenic structure.

<u>V. Moennig</u> I was not thinking of just one monoclonal antibody,
but of a whole group of antibodies, so that you test each antibody on the isolate and thus differentiate the strains.

<u>J. Asso</u> *(France)* Is it possible to imagine that several
glycoproteins play a role as a neutralising site?

<u>G. Pauli</u> It certainly is but, if there are two or three
glycoproteins in one precipitation band, we cannot decide, by
the methods we use at present, whether all three are involved
or only one of them; nor do we know what role it plays. It may

be that one glycoprotein is involved in direct neutralisation whilst the other one is involved in neutralisation through complement. In another system, when we compared HSV-1 and BHN virus, we found you can divide it into two sites, one site is involved directly in neutralisation and the other is involved through complement. So you can say that you have different glycoproteins which play different roles during the infection.

J. Asso   But my point is that maybe the antigenic sites for neutralisation are made by different glycoproteins and that you destroy them. So, when you do this kind of analysis you are playing with proteins which are separated from each other.

G. Pauli   But in a case where you have the antiserum against one protein, and the antiserum is neutralised, then you know that you have recognised the right site. If it is not neutralising, then you are not sure whether or not it is due to an unfolding during the preparation. If you have a positive result, then all is clear.

H. Ludwig   With all viruses you have to separate the components to study the analyses and then maybe do a synthesis. We know by using immune electronmicroscopy in other systems that antibodies directed against those precipitates still recognise the intact site on the virions. The possibility exists that some antigens together form an important site but the problem is how to test it.

K. Dalsgaard   (Denmark)   This 80 kilodalton glycoprotein you are talking about as definitely having something to do with neutralisation: does it appear early in the replication cycle and does it stay as an 80 kilodalton protein all the way through?

G. Pauli   We did not test that.

K. Dalsgaard   When was it demonstrated as an 80 kilodalton protein?

G. Pauli   About 20 hours post infection, and we labelled between 5 hours and 20 hours post infection.

G. Wittmann   (Federal Republic of Germany)   Of how many proteins does the Aujeszky's virus consist?

G. Pauli   Between 20 and 30. It is similar to the other herpes viruses. Also with the immunogenic components, there is not much difference with the other herpes viruses.

H. Ludwig   Some years ago, Stevely in Glasgow analysed purified ADV and he found 27 or so structural proteins. Of course it is true that if you look for the infected cell proteins it will be around 40 or 50 and maybe those infected cell proteins might play a major role in immune defence. That field is completely open for research.

M. Pensaert (Belgium)   What is the situation these days: is anyone working with DNA recombinants for production of antigens in ADV?

H. Ludwig   I don't know of any small scientific groups, but I am convinced that the Biogene laboratory in Switzerland and the American laboratories are working on it. But I think the question is to know what you should clone. It is ridiculous to clone the whole genome at the moment.

A.L.J. Gielkens   Yes, that is too complex of course.

H. Ludwig   I think we must be a little critical of just cloning DNA for fun - wasting money and brains simply to do something in the scientific field because it can be done. We must know the basis first.

CHARACTERISTICS OF FIELD AND MODIFIED AUJESZKY'S DISEASE VIRUS STRAINS

F. Tozzini

Istituto di Malattie Infettive,
Facoltà Veterinaria, 56100 Pisa, Italy.

ABSTRACT

Four Aujeszky's disease virus strains isolated from pigs, the live vaccine used in Italy and an experimental modified strain, were character-ised by their behaviour in tissue culture, their thermal sensitivity and rabbit virulence markers. Significant reduction of titre and plaque size was observed when the vaccine strain which was adapted to grow on chicken embryo fibroblasts was titrated on RK13 cells. Heat sensitivity ranged from the heat resistant experimental modified strain, to the less resistant vaccine strain, to the heat sensitive field strains. Using the rabbit virulence test no differences were observed between the vaccine strain and the four field isolated strains; in all cases the rabbits died with pruritus within three days. The experimental modified strain killed almost all the inoculated animals but the survival time was prolonged to 6 - 9 days and there were fewer cases of pruritus.

INTRODUCTION

The use of live vaccines to control Aujeszky's disease (AD) in swine in Europe has created the need for reliable means of differentiating field Aujeszky's disease virus (ADV) from the vaccinal strains. Effective and practical means of differ-entiation are important for epidemiological research in swine but also for when cases of AD are reported in animals of other species. The exact identification of a vaccinal strain would be of particular interest in Italy where a live vaccine is used in the field to control swine AD and where a high number of swine are arriving for slaughter from the European Community countries and from eastern Europe.

In this paper we report the results of a characterisation study conducted on six AD strains. Some cultural aspects, the heat sensitivity and the rabbit virulence of these strains have been considered.

G. Wittmann, S.A. Hall (eds), Aujeszky's Disease. ISBN-13:978-94-009-7555-2

MATERIALS AND METHODS

Cells

The RK13 cell line and secondary chicken embryo fibroblasts (CEF) were used. The cultures were prepared on Nunclon plastic or on glass containers (24 cm^2). Growth and maintenance medium consisted of 199 with 10% newborn calf serum, gentamycin sulphate plus mycostatin and 0.2% $NaHCO_3$. When the plaque method was used the maintenance medium contained 1.2% of Bacto Agar.

Viruses

The origin and history of the viruses used are the following: 1) Strain Pisa 80, isolated on RK13 cells from the brain of a pig; 2) Strain Leghorn 78, isolated on PK15 cells from the tonsil of a pig slaughtered under normal conditions; 3) Strain Siena 79, isolated on RK13 cells from the brain of a pig; 4) Strain Grosseto 80, isolated on RK13 cells from the brain of a pig; 5) Live commercial vaccine, produced by Istituto Zooprofilattico, Brescia (Vaccine BS), with an unknown number of passages on chicken embryo fibroblasts. 6) Strain modified T, originated from the live vaccine BS, serially passaged at $30^{\circ}C$ on RK13 cells. Every four passages the virus suspension was heated at $50^{\circ}C$ for 60 min. After 18 passages the virus was heated at $56^{\circ}C$ for 30 min and cultured on RK13 cells at $30^{\circ}C$ where a plaque of virus developed after 10 days; the 20th passage was then made.

The strains from 1 to 5 were passaged once on RK13 cells before being used in the tests.

Virus assay

There are several reports in the literature (in Lautie, 1967; Majer Dziedzic, 1979) on the behaviour of vaccinal and virulent AD strains on tissue cultures and on the size of plaques produced.

Confluent cell cultures were infected by replacing the culture medium with dilutions of the virus suspensions (0.1 ml) and leaving them for 30 min at $37^{\circ}C$ for adsorption. The medium

was then replaced and the cultures were held at 37°C for one
week and examined twice a day for CPE or plaque recordings.
Titres were expressed as PFU/ml or $TCID_{50}$/ml.

Heat Sensitivity

Heat resistance has been indicated by Bodon et al. (1968)
and by Bartha et al. (1969) as a marker of reduced virulence of
the ADV strain. Platt et al. (1979) studying field and vaccinal
strains have observed marked differences among the field strains
and also between the K and BUK vaccines examined.

Toma (1979) and Toma et al. (1979) have selected a vaccinal
strain by serial passage at low temperature. The growth of this
strain is thermosensitive.

Virus suspensions diluted to a titre of $10^{3.5} TCID_{50}$/0.1 ml,
were incubated in a 50°C water bath for 30 min. After incubation
serial tenfold dilutions were made and each dilution inoculated
into four RK13 cultures. The titres were recorded one week
later. Unheated suspensions were also titrated to determine the
original titre. The experiment was repeated one week later.
Any dilution was made with maintenance medium.

Studies in rabbits

The recent experiences of Platt et al. (1979) have shown
that the rabbit virulence test is the most useful test for
differentiating between vaccinal and virulent strains.

Strains of virus were compared in rabbits (New Zealand
weighing 2 - 3 kg) by their ability to cause pruritus and by the
time required to kill. Rabbits were divided into groups and
inoculated subcutaneously in the right costal region with one ml
of virus suspension previously diluted with medium to contain
10^4 $TCID_{50}$. The rabbits were then observed twice a day for signs
of infection and death.

RESULTS

1) Cultural characteristics

The plaque forming characteristics of the four field
strains and the modified T strain were identical in RK13 cells
and CEF cells. The vaccine BS strain was markedly different;
in RK13 cells the titre was significantly reduced and the size
of the plaques after four days incubation was half that of the
other strains. On CEF cells the diameter of the plaques was
the same for all six strains examined (Table 1).

TABLE 1

INFECTIOUS TITRES AND DIAMETER OF PLAQUES (IN BRACKETS) IN TISSUE CULTURES

Strain	On RK13	On CEF
1 Field isolate	32×10^3 (2)*	30×10^3 (3)
2 " "	24×10^3 (2)	22×10^3 (3)
3 " "	30×10^3 (2)	28×10^3 (3)
4 " "	22×10^3 (2)	25×10^3 (3)
5 Vaccine BS	40×10^2 (1)	30×10^3 (3)
6 Modified T	28×10^3 (2)	32×10^3 (3)

* Diameter in mm

2) Heat sensitivity

The results of our experiments reported in Table 2
indicate a difference in heat sensitivity among the strains
used. The four field strains presented a reduction in titre
of 3 log when heated at 50°C. This difference was of 2 log
for the vaccine BS and of 0.5 log for the modified T, indicating a heat resistance increasing with the grade of attenuation.

3) Rabbit virulence

In our virulence tests the results (Table 3) indicated
no difference between the vaccine strain and the field isolates.
Each one induced pruritus and death within 3 days.

TABLE 2

HEAT SENSITIVITY OF AUJESZKY'S DISEASE VIRUS STRAIÑS.   TITRES (RECIPROCAL LOG 10)

Strain	Before heating	After heating	Difference
1 Field isolate	3.5	0.5	3.0
2 " "	3.5	0.5	3.0
3 " "	3.5	0.5	3.0
4 " "	3.5	0.5	3.0
5 Vaccine BS	3.5	1.5	2.0
6 Modified T	3.5	3.0	0.5

TABLE 3

COMPARISON OF AUJESZKY'S DISEASE VIRUSES AS MEASURED BY VIRULENCE FOR RABBITS

Strain	Rabbits inoculated	% pruritus	% mortality	Survival time (in days)
1 Field isolate	8	100	100	3
2 " "	6	100	100	3
3 " "	6	100	100	3
4 " "	6	100	100	3
5 Vaccine BS	8	100	100	3
6 Modified T	12	54.5	91	6 - 9

A substantial difference was observed with the modified T strain. Although it was lethal for rabbits they survived longer and there were fewer cases of pruritus.

CONCLUSIONS

The rabbit virulence test must be considered unsuitable to identify the live vaccine used in Italy. The comparative titrations conducted on different substrates and the heat sensitivity test could help in the identification of the vaccine strain if further studies confirm that these characteristics are stable after passage of the virus in the pig. The tests conducted on the experimentally modified T strain which originated from the vaccine BS, have shown that the modification has induced interesting markers of heat sensitivity and rabbit virulence. Further studies are also necessary in this case to verify these markers after passages in pig and to control the characteristics of antigenicity.

REFERENCES

Bartha, A., Belak, S. and Benyeda, J., 1969. Trypsin and heat resistance of some strains of the herpesvirus group. Acta Vet. Acad. Sc. Hung., 19, 97-99.
Bodon, L., Meszaros, J., Papp-Vid, G. and Romvary, J., 1968. Properties of Aujeszky's disease virus strains isolated from swine pneumonia cases. Act. Vet. Acad. Sc. Hung. 18, 107-109.
Lautie, R., 1969. La maladie d'Aujeszky. Expens. Scient. Franc.
Majer-Dziedzic, B., 1979. Genetic properties of selected strains of the Aujeszky disease virus. Polsk. Arch. Weter. 21, 41-49.
Platt, K.B., Mare, C.J. and Hinz, P.N., 1979. Differentiation of vaccine strains and field isolates of pseudorabies virus: thermal sensitivity and rabbit virulence markers. Arch. of Vir. 60, 13, 23.
Toma, B., 1979. Obtention et caracterisation d'une souche thermosensible de virus de la maladie d'Aujeszky (souche Alfort 26). Rec. Med. Vet. 155, 131-137.
Toma, B., Brun, A., Chappuis, G. and Terze, J., 1979. Propriétés biologiques d'une souche thermosensible (Alfort 26) de virus de la maladie d'Aujeszky. Rec. Med. Vet. 155, 245-252.

DISCUSSION

H. Ludwig *(Federal Republic of Germany)* Do you have any strains which at a dose level of, say, 1 000 plaque forming units, do not kill rabbits?

F. Tozzini *(Italy)* No, we do not have such a strain. All the field strains kill the rabbits in three days. The rabbit is very sensitive.

J.B. McFerran *(UK)* The NIA-4 strain does not kill rabbits.

B. Toma *(France)* I don't think the Bartha strain kills rabbits either.

J.B. McFerran It does sometimes but not always. Mostly it does not.

F. Tozzini I believe the K strain is not pathogenic for rabbits.

H. Ludwig   Dr. McFerran, how do you inoculate the rabbit with the Bartha strain to kill or not to kill it, intra-muscularly or intra-peritoneally?

J.B. McFerran   There seems to be no reason to it. You can inoculate five rabbits intra-muscularly and they will all live; you can do it again and one will die, even though the dose is the same.

H. Ludwig   I asked because the route of infection I think is an important factor in whether or not it kills. I think that if you choose the right route and give the immune response a chance with a low virulent strain, it might get the virus somewhere. That was the basis for my question.

F. Tozzini   With our modified D strain, designated for the vaccine BAS we inoculated 12 rabbits and we had a mortality of 91% with pruritus in 54%, but in that case the time factor was important. The rabbits died in six to nine days - it was a longer time.

H. Ludwig   Maybe they died by immune response.

J.Th. van Oirschot (Netherlands) Do you use these modified live vaccine strains in the field?

F. Tozzini   No, we have not done that. It is still at the experimental stage.

SESSION II

DIAGNOSTIC PROCEDURES

Chairman: B. Toma

COMPLEMENT-DEPENDENT NEUTRALISATION OF AUJESZKY'S DISEASE VIRUS BY ANTIBODY

V. Bitsch[1] and M. Eskildsen[2]

[1] State Veterinary Serum Laboratory, Bulowsvej 27, DK-1870 Copenhagen V, Denmark.
[2] State Veterinary Institute for Virus Research, Lindholm, DK-4771 Kalvehave, Denmark.

ABSTRACT

The complement-dependent neutralisation reaction in tests for demonstration of Aujeszky's disease virus-neutralising antibody (VNA) was studied. Guinea pig serum was the source of complement (C') and the concentrations giving optimum augmentation of antibody titres were determined. Both IgM and IgG contained C'-requiring VNA. IgM antibody produced early in the course of immunisation showed the highest degree of C'-dependency, while no difference in this respect could be found between early and late IgG antibody. Appropriate concentrations of C' enhanced IgM antibody titres by up to 9 $\log_2$ units and raised IgG antibody titres 3 to 4 $\log_2$ units. A linear relationship was demonstrated between C'-enhanced VNA titres and the preincubation period. C' was found to act only on preformed infectious virus-antibody complexes, and the full effect could be achieved by adding C' to the virus-serum mixtures a relatively short time before inoculation of cell cultures. Addition of C' to the virus-serum mixtures at the beginning of preincubation gave reduced enhancement of VNA titres.

INTRODUCTION

Infectious virus-antibody complexes are formed with a variety of viruses. Such virus-antibody complexes can be rendered non-infectious by complement (Yoshino and Taniguchi, 1964) or anti-immunoglobulins (Ashe and Notkins, 1966). Although several papers have demonstrated that complement-requiring neutralising antibody is produced in animals infected with Aujeszky's disease virus (ADV), a more detailed investigation of the complement-dependent neutralisation reaction in the Aujeszky's disease (AD) virus-neutralising antibody (VNA) test does not seem to have been performed. The present study was initiated in an effort to supply this want.

MATERIALS AND METHODS

Sera

The samples were collected from experimental pigs infected

G. Wittmann, S.A. Hall (eds), Aujeszky's Disease. ISBN-13:978-94-009-7555-2

nasally with Danish strains of ADV. In one experiment, however, sera from naturally infected pigs were used. For reduction and inactivation of IgM, sera were treated with 2-mercaptoethanol (2-MC) as described by Eskildsen (1975). IgG and IgM were pre-pared as described by Metzger and Fougereau (1967) and Curtis and Bourne (1971), respectively.

VNA tests

The virus strain DaS67 and primary pig kidney or primary or secondary pig testis cell monolayers in tissue culture tubes were used. Maintenance medium was Eagle's minimal essential medium with 2% heat-inactivated bovine serum. Hanks' salt solution with 2% serum as above was used for virus suspensions and serum dilutions.

All sera were heat-inactivated at $56^{\circ}C$. Incubation of virus-serum mixtures (preincubation) was performed at $37^{\circ}C$ for 24 h (P37/24 test) if not mentioned otherwise. Two or 4 cul-tures, in one case 6, were inoculated from each virus-serum mixture, each culture receiving 0.2 ml. When guinea pig serum was added, the inoculation dose was increased proportionally.

Guinea pig serum stored at $-55^{\circ}C$ served as a source of complement (C'). Three different pools were used, which con-tained from 45 to 56 100% haemolytic units per 0.1 ml. Unless otherwise mentioned, C' was added to the virus-serum mixtures 45 to 60 min before inoculation.

More details are given in the description of individual experiments.

CF test

Sera from naturally infected pigs were tested by a modified direct complement fixation test, performed as described by Eskildsen (1975).

EXPERIMENTS AND RESULTS

Experiment 1. The effect of the concentration of C' on neutralisation

Early convalescent-phase sera were used: untreated sera

taken from one pig on days 13 and 15 p.i. and 2-MC-treated sera
taken from another pig on days 20 and 48 p.i. Previously, the
VNA titres of untreated/2-MC-treated sera from days 20 and 48
had been found to be 720/90 and 720/360, respectively. Titres
of the 2-MC-treated sera from days 13 and 15 were < 2.

A twofold dilution series was prepared from the guinea
pig serum that served as source of C'. Titrations of the sera
were performed with each of these C' dilutions, each time by
adding the same amount of C' dilution to the virus-serum mixtures. Four cultures were inoculated from each mixture except
in one case (13-day serum), where 6 cultures were used. Control
titrations with heat-inactivated C' were included.

IgG and IgM from early immune serum were tested similarly.
VNA titres of 2 and 4.8, respectively, had been recorded for
these preparations. Two cultures were inoculated from each
dilution.

Results are shown in Figures 1a and 1b.

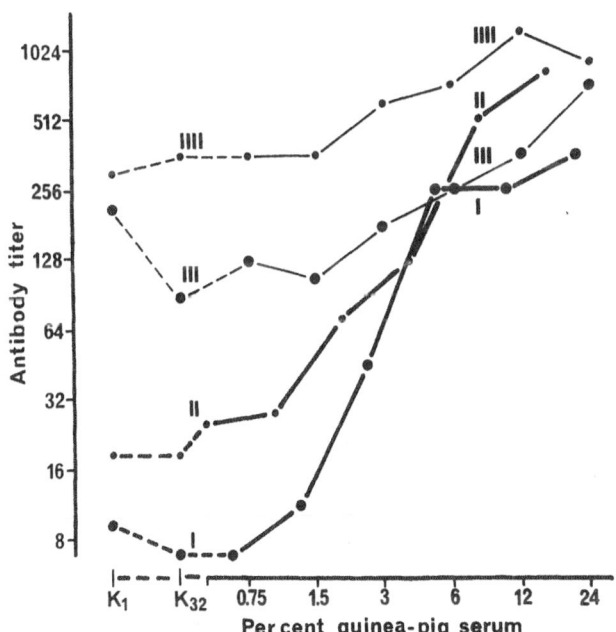

Fig. 1a. The relationships between concentration of complement and VNA
titres of untreated and 2-MC-treated sera from the early convalescent phase. I, II: untreated sera from days 13 (I) and 15 (II) p.i.
III, IIII: 2-MC-treated sera from days 20 (III) and 48 (IIII) p.i.
K_1, K_{32}: heat-inactivated complement used undiluted (K_1) and diluted
1:32 (K_{32}).

44

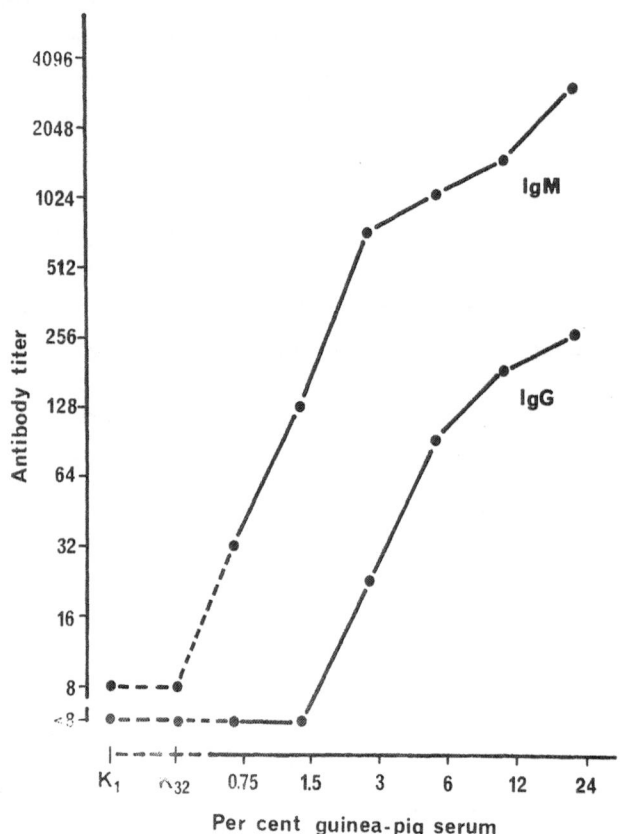

Fig. 1b. The relationships between concentration of complement and VNA
titres of IgM and IgG from early convalescent-phase serum.
K_1, K_{32}: see explanation to Figure 1a.

Experiment 2. The effect of C' in excess on the progression of the C'-dependent neutralisation

Early convalescent-phase serum collected 13 days p.i. was
used. A VNA test dilution series was prepared from the serum
and preincubated at 37°C for 24 h. At the start of incubation
and after 5, 11 and 23 h aliquots were taken from each virus-
serum mixture for addition of 9% C', after which they were again
placed at 37°C. Titres were determined for all these dilution
series after 3, 6, 12 and 24 h as calculated from the beginning
of preincubation for the original dilution series. A control
titration with heat-inactivated C' added at the start of

preincubation was included.   Four cultures were inoculated from
each dilution.

Results are given in Figure 2.

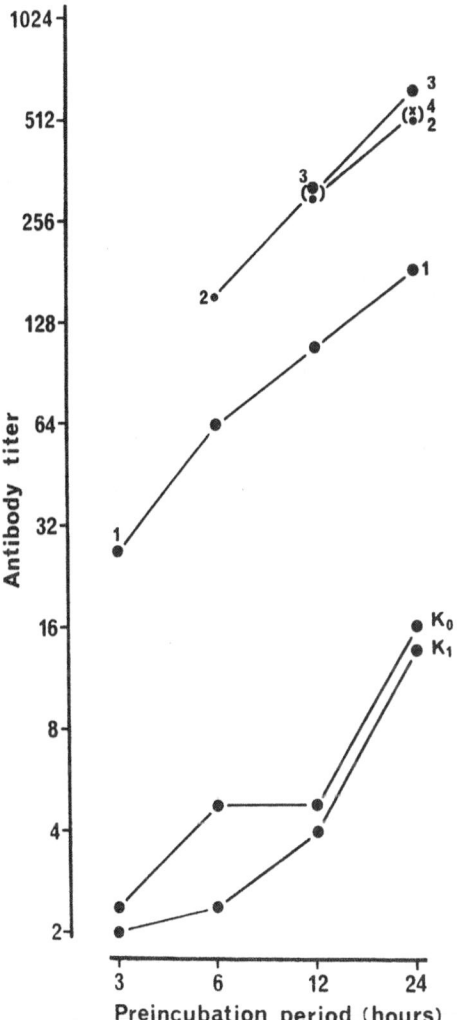

Fig. 2.   The effect of complement in excess on the progression of complement-
dependent neutralisation.
K_O, K_1: titres when no complement (K_O) and heat-inactivated
complement (K_1) was added.
1-1, 2-2, 3-3, 4: complement added at the start of preincubation
and after 5, 11 and 23 h, respectively.

46

Experiment 3. The development of C'-requiring and non-C'-requiring VNA during the acute-infection phase and early convalescent phase

Serum was taken daily from a nasally infected pig and tested untreated and 2-MC-treated, in both cases with and without addition of C' (15%). Two cultures were inoculated from each dilution.

The results are shown in Figure 3.

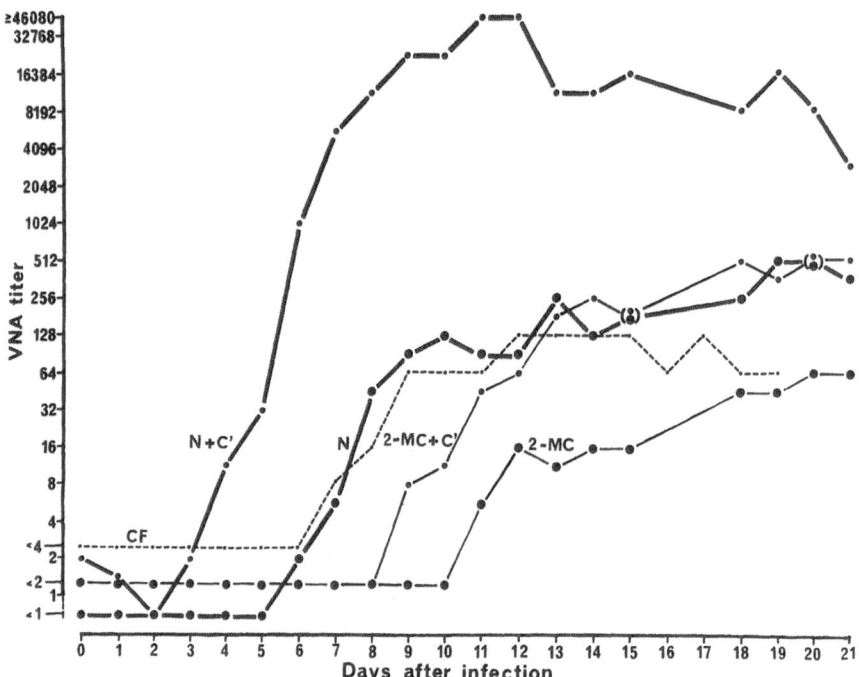

Fig. 3. The development of complement-requiring and non-complement-requiring VNA in serum of a nasally infected pig during the acute infection and early convalescent phase.
N, N + C': titres of untreated sera before and after addition of complement, respectively.
2-MC, 2-MC + C': titres of 2-MC-treated sera before and after addition of complement, respectively.
CF: complement-fixing antibody titres.

Experiment 4. The presence of C'-requiring and non-C'-requiring VNA in late convalescent-phase sera

Sera from 24 pigs known to have become naturally infected

approximately two years prior to the sampling were tested as
described for Experiment 3.

The results are shown in Figure 4. The mean titre
improvement after addition of C' was 3.4 $\log_2$ units for untreated
sera and 3.5 $\log_2$ units for 2-MC-treated sera.

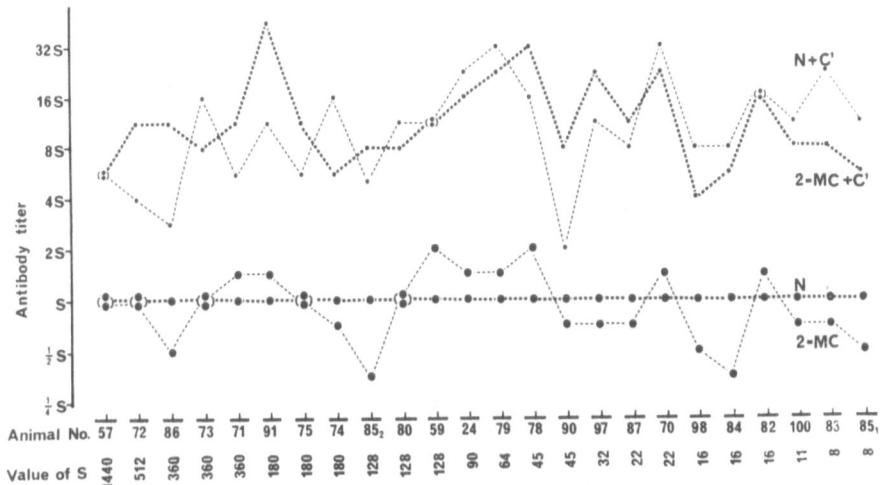

Fig. 4. Titres of complement-requiring and non-complement-requiring VNA in
late convalescent-phase serum of 24 naturally infected pigs.
Symbols, see explanations to Figure 3.

DISCUSSION AND CONCLUSIONS

Since treatment of serum with 2-MC will result in decom-
position of IgM and inhibition of its neutralising effect, but
will leave IgG unchanged, both Figures 1a and 1b demonstrate
that early IgG as well as IgM contains C'-requiring VNA. Six
to 10% of the pool of guinea pig serum that served as source of
C' appear to give optimum neutralisation by IgM, whereas slightly higher concentrations would seem to be required by IgG. In
this respect it should be borne in mind that the neutralisation-
enhancing effect of C' is proportional to its haemolytical activity (Taniguchi and Yoshino, 1965).

Two important conclusions can be drawn from Experiment 2.
Firstly, the progression of neutralisation by C'-requiring VNA
in a VNA test proceeds linearly with time (linear relationship
between VNA titre and preincubation period, see Figure 2), which

is in full accordance with the lines that have been demonstrated for non-C'-dependent neutralisation (Bitsch, 1978). The somewhat irregular course of the control neutralisation curves (K_0 and K_1) is in keeping with personal experience, in that a sharp neutralisation endpoint cannot usually be obtained with early convalescent-phase serum. This phenomenon is probably caused by interference from the C'-requiring IgM antibody present in high concentration. Secondly, C' has no effect on the rate of union between virus and antibody. It acts only on preformed infectious virus-antibody complexes, and neutralisation occurs rapidly. In assays not shown here (authors' unpublished material) the full effect was seen when C' in excess was added as late as 5 to 10 min before inoculation.

It is also worth noticing that even after early addition of C', e.g. after 5 h at 37°C, an effect could be seen on virus-antibody combinations formed many hours later. A reduced enhancement of neutralisation, however, was seen, when C' was added at the start of preincubation. An identical observation has been made by Rossi and Kiesel (1976) who, in P37/2 tests for VNA to infectious bovine rhinotracheitis virus, compared addition at the beginning of preincubation with addition after 1 h.

Incorporation of C' in a P37/24 VNA test resulted in demonstration of antibody as early as 4 days after nasal infection, and extremely high titres could be demonstrated a few days later, titre enhancements by C' being up to 9 $\log_2$ units (Figure 3). This illustrates the fact that a test modified by addition of complement will be extremely sensitive for demonstration of early VNA (IgM). However, neutralisation by IgG in sera from long after infection will also be enhanced by C' (Figure 4). The unexpectedly high improvement of 3 to 4 $\log_2$ units is probably related to the high concentration of C' used and the fact that C' was added late during the preincubation, i.e. about 45 min before inoculation.

It was surprising that the CF test demonstrated antibody earlier than the ordinary VNA test used on the same 2-MC-treated sera, although the CF and VNA titres in sera taken relatively few days later were almost identical. This would seem to

indicate that the CF reaction with sera from the early immunisation phase is more complex than with sera from later periods.

In conclusion, a VNA test modified by incorporation of C'
is an extremely sensitive tool for demonstration of early IgM
antibody to ADV. The enhancement of the neutralisation by IgG
in late convalescent-phase sera is also considerable. To obtain
high sensitivity, a P37/24 test or a modification possessing a
corresponding or even higher sensitivity should preferably be
employed. The appropriate amount of C' should be added late,
e.g. 30 min prior to the inoculation.

REFERENCES

Ashe, W.K. and Notkins, A.L., 1966. Neutralization of an infectious herpes
    simplex virus-antibody complex by anti-γ-globulin. Proc. Nat. Acid.
    Sci., 56, 447-451.
Bitsch, V., 1978. An investigation into the basic virus-antibody neutral-
    ization reaction, with special regard to the reaction in the constant-
    virus/varying-serum neutralization test. Acta. Vet. Scand., 19,
    110-128.
Curtis, J. and Bourne, F.J., 1971. Immunoglobulin quantitation in sow serum,
    colostrum and milk and the serum of young pigs. Biochem. Biophys.
    Acta (Amst.), 236, 319-332.
Eskildsen, M., 1975. Demonstration of antibodies against pseudorabies virus
    in swine serum by a modified direct complement fixation test. Bull.
    Off. Int. Epiz., 84, 253-263.
Metzger, J.J. and Fougereau, M., 1967. Caracterisation de deux sous-
    classes d'immunoglobulines γ G chez le porc. C.R. Acad. Sci. (Paris),
    265, 724-727.
Rossi, C.R. and Kiesel, G.K., 1976. Antibody class and complement require-
    ment of neutralizing antibodies in the primary and secondary antibody
    response of cattle to infectious bovine rhinotracheitis virus vaccine.
    Arch. Virology, 51, 191-198.
Taniguchi, S. and Yoshino, K., 1965. Studies on the neutralization of
    herpes simplex virus. II Analysis of complement as the antibody-
    potentiating factor. Virology, 26, 54-60.
Yoshino, K. and Taniguchi, S., 1964. The appearance of complement-
    requiring neutralizing antibodies by immunization and infection with
    herpes simplex virus. Virology, 22, 193-201.

COMPARATIVE EVALUATION OF 'ELISA' AND NEUTRALISATION TEST FOR THE DIAGNOSIS OF AUJESZKY'S DISEASE

V. Moennig[1], P. Woldesenbet[1], H.-R. Frey[1], B. Liess[1],
H.D. Dopatka[2] and F. Behrens[2]

[1] Institute for Virology, Veterinary School,
Bischofsholer Damm 15, D-3000 Hannover 1,

[2] Behringwerke, D-3550 Marburg 1,
Federal Republic of Germany.

INTRODUCTION

In recent years a rising incidence of Aujeszky's disease in pigs has been reported in the north-western districts and other parts of Germany (Bee and Frost, 1981). Both the farming industry and veterinary authorities are particularly concerned at the possibility of a further spread of the disease. The identification of antibody carriers in infected breeding herds and their elimination are promising ways of handling the present situation. Since this would require facilities for a large scale serological investigation, there has been an increasing interest in laboratory techniques for the detection of antibody against Aujeszky's disease virus (ADV). Some investigators have tried to establish the enzyme-linked immunosorbent assay (ELISA) for the detection of ADV-antibodies in pigs (Moutou et al., 1978; Briaire et al., 1979). Compared to the conventional serum neutralisation test (SNT) the ELISA would offer some advantages for the screening of large numbers of sera. However, at present there are only a few reports published on its specificity, sensitivity and reproducibility in field diagnosis (Forschner et al., 1981). In the present study 471 porcine field sera were investigated using a commercially available ELISA (Enzygnost, Behringwerke) and a SNT. Furthermore both tests were compared in seven animals which were experimentally infected with ADV.

EXPERIMENTAL STUDY

For kinetic studies seven piglets, aged about three weeks, were inoculated intranasally with 3 000 infectious units of ADV each. Between the 5th and 7th day p.i. all animals showed a

moderate temperature rise. Blood samples were taken five times
at intervals of three days. Thereafter the animals were bled
weekly for another six weeks. Sera were tested in the SNT and
in the ELISA. The SNT was performed on PK(15) cells using the
microtitre system. Minimal serum dilutions started at 1 : 2.
No extra complement was added to the samples. The ELISA method
is illustrated in Figure 1. For screening purposes sera were
diluted 1 : 20 and 1 : 80. They were tested on ADV-antigen as
well as on a negative control antigen. Antibodies were detected
using a phosphatase-coupled antiserum against pig IgG. A difference in optical density at 405 nm of more than 0.2 units between
antigen well and control well was considered to be positive. In
general the results showed a good correlation between the tests
(Figure 2). However, in four out of seven piglets the ELISA
seemed to be more sensitive and detected ADV-antibodies a few
days earlier than the SN test. Relatively high ELISA titres
ranging from 1 : 160 to 1 : 320 were observed on the tenth day
after infection. A fifth animal showed a doubtful ELISA titre
of 1 : 20. At that time no significant neutralising activity

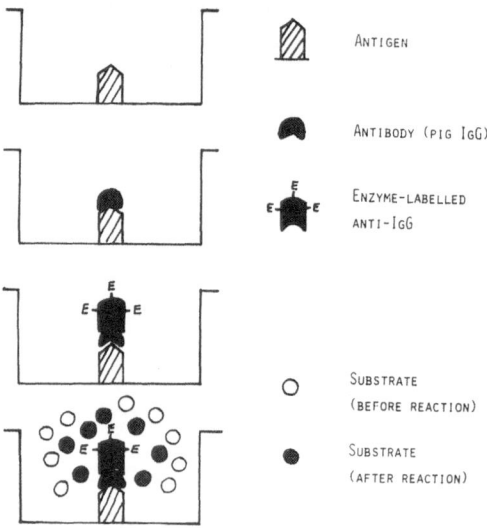

Fig. 1. Enzyme-linked immunosorbent assay (ELISA) for the detection of
Aujeszky virus-specific antibodies in porcine sera.

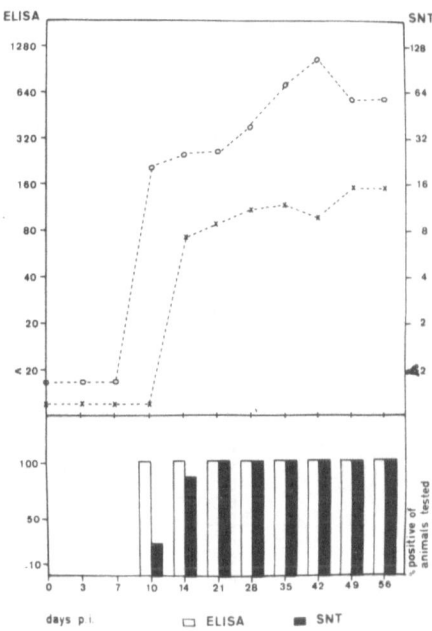

Fig. 2. Development of Aujeszky virus-specific antibodies after
experimental infection of pigs.

was detectable. Only four days later all but one serum sample
were positive in the SNT. This drawback of the SNT is probably
due to the fact that no complement was used in the test. The
addition of complement is reported to enhance the sensitivity
of the SNT and antibody detection is possible as early as on
the seventh day p.i. (Wittmann, 1981).

FIELD STUDY

In a second study 471 porcine field sera from several
herds from the north-western part of Lower Saxony were investigated using both test systems. Out of 51 herds, 35 herds were

anamnestically suspected to have Aujeszky's disease (AD) and
the remaining 16 randomised herds had no special anamnesis.
The results of a screening test are summarised in Table 1.
Five sera were not evaluated in the SNT because they were toxic
for the cells. Discrepancies were observed in eight cases, which
is an accordance of 97.2%. Six sera reacted negatively in the
SNT and positively in the ELISA. Five of these sera came from
four herds with an AD anamnesis. Two sera were negative in the
ELISA but positive in the SNT. One serum originated from the
group of herds suspected to have AD and the other from the un-
suspected herds. A closer look at these eight results shows
that, with one exception, positive reactions were only observed
in the lowest serum dilution. In only one of these cases an
ELISA titre of 1 : 40 versus a negative SN was registered.

TABLE 1

RESULTS OF A COMPARATIVE SCREENING TEST OF 471 PORCINE FIELD SERA

		ELISA	
		Positive	Negative
SNT	Positive	158	2
	Negative	6	300
	Toxic	1	4
Total: 471 Sera			

Positive sera were then titrated and results were compared.
Although ELISA titres were considerably higher than SNT titres
the titration curves corresponded well. The results are shown
in Figure 3. Considering the different anamnestic situation of
the herds it became clear that the significance of the clinical
anamnesis was irrelevant. In both groups about 60% of the
herds were seronegative versus about 40% seropositive ones.

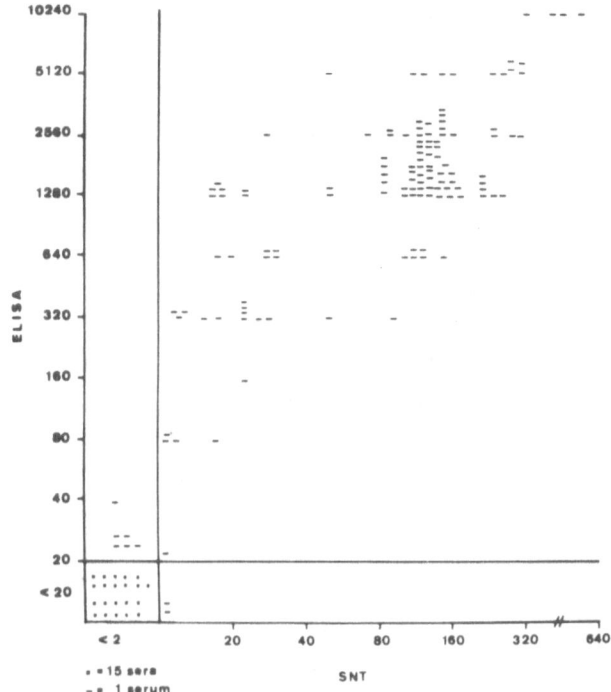

Fig. 3. Comparison of ELISA and SNT titres of 132 ADV positive field sera.

DISCUSSION

Our discovery that the comparison of a larger group of sera will yield more positive samples in the ELISA system was predictable considering the outcome of our first serological investigation. The high sensitivity of the ELISA explains the higher number of positive sera detected by this test. The existence of toxic sera is also a fact. Since the ELISA does not depend on cultured cells these sera are not lost to a serological survey. However we have no convincing explanation for the second group of sera, which reacted positively in the SNT but negatively in the ELISA. Possibly these sera contained low amounts of virus-inhibiting substances other than immunoglobulins, since no cross-reactions with other viruses occurring in pigs are known so far. The titration of the field sera

confirmed the results obtained from our first experiment.
Titration curves were parallel to each other, ELISA titres
being higher than SNT titres.

Our experiments led us to the conclusion that the ELISA
for the detection of antibodies against ADV may be a useful tool
for performing large scale serological investigations. Compared
with the standard SNT the ELISA shows a slightly higher sensitivity, a good reproducibility and a high specificity. In addition this test offers advantages from the point of view of the
laboratory since it does not require cultured cells.

ACKNOWLEDGEMENTS

The authors wish to thank Professor Dr. Reuss and Dr.
Bechmann for the generous supply of field sera.

REFERENCES

Bee, A.H. and Frost, J.W., 1981. Serologische Untersuchungen über die
  Häufigkeit und Verbreitung neutralisierender Antikörper gegen das
  Virus der Aujeszkyschen Krankheit bei Schweinen in Hessen.
  Dtsch. Tierärztl. Wschr. 88, 168-169.
Briaire, J., Meloen, R.H. and Barteling, J.S., 1979. An enzyme-linked
  immunosorbent assay (ELISA) for the detection of antibody against
  Aujeszky's disease virus in pig sera. Zbl. Vet. Med. B 26, 76-81.
Forschner, E., Dopatka, H.D., Buenger, I., Behrens, F. and Witte, K.H.,
  1981. Aujeszkysche Krankheit des Schweines: Zur Einsatzmöglichkeit
  eines ELISAs für den Nachweis von virusspezifischen Serumantikörpern.
  Dtsch. Tierärztl. Wschr. 88, 134-139.
Moutou, F., Toma, B. and Fortier, B., 1978. Application of an enzyme-
  linked immunosorbent assay for diagnosis of Aujeszky's disease in
  swine. Vet. Rec., 102, 264.
Wittmann, G., 1981. personal communication.

INFLUENCE OF VACCINATION WITH MODIFIED LIVE VACCINE ON THE LABORATORY DIAGNOSIS OF AUJESZKY'S DISEASE

C. Terpstra and J.M.A. Pol

Central Veterinary Institute, Virology Department,
Houtribweg 39, 8221 RA Lelystad, The Netherlands.

ABSTRACT

Litters of two week-old piglets were vaccinated with commercially available modified live virus (MLV) vaccines and killed at intervals between 4 and 14 days post vaccination. Parts of the central nervous system, tonsils and lungs were collected for virus isolation and for immunofluorescent and histopathologic studies. No virus, viral antigen or histopathologic lesions were detected after vaccination with strain MK-25. However, small quantities of Aujeszky's disease virus (ADV) were recovered on the fourth day after vaccination with the Ayvak strain. An erroneous diagnosis of Aujeszky's Disease (AD) as a result of the use of MLV vaccines therefore seems unlikely when histopathologic or immunofluorescent methods are employed. Histopathological lesions in the central nervous system of two control piglets inoculated with virulent ADV were inconsistent with the severity of the clinical signs, course of disease and virus titres.

INTRODUCTION

Modified live virus (MLV) vaccines are used in various Eastern and Western European countries, and in the USA to control Aujeszky's disease (AD) in pigs. Replication of the vaccine virus in the host is a prerequisite for a MLV vaccine to provoke an immune response. De Leeuw and Tiessink (1980) have shown that several commercial MLV vaccines against AD may give rise to shedding of vaccine virus from the oral or nasal cavity. The spread of virus from the site of inoculation to other parts of the body could also interfere with the laboratory diagnosis of AD.

The purpose of the present work was to investigate the chances of misinterpreting results of laboratory diagnostic tests, after a previous vaccination against AD with two MLV vaccines that are widely used in the Netherlands.

G. Wittmann, S.A. Hall (eds), Aujeszky's Disease. ISBN-13:978-94-009-7555-2

MATERIALS AND METHODS

Vaccines and virus strains

Two commercial vaccines*, both produced on chick embryo
fibroblast cultures, were investigated. The virulent Northern
Ireland Aujeszky 3 (NIA-3) strain was used to infect control
piglets. A plaque titration in pig kidney cell cultures was
performed on a portion of each inoculum.

Experimental animals

Piglets of the Dutch landrace were obtained from the
Institute's farm, which has no history of AD. Two litters of
eight piglets were vaccinated at two weeks old with one of the
vaccine strains. Vaccines were applied in accordance with the
instructions of the producers, each animal receiving a dose of
2 ml by the intramuscular route. Another two piglets aged
4 weeks received strain NIA-3 intramuscularly into the neck and
served as controls.

Collection and preparation of samples

At 4, 7, 10 and 14 days post vaccination, two piglets were
slaughtered and subjected to a systematic autopsy, using separate sterile instruments to collect the tissues. The control
pigs were autopsied at 4 days post inoculation. The tissues
that were collected are listed in Tables 1 and 2. Samples for
virus isolation were placed in sterile capped universals of
known weight, whereas samples intended for sectioning were snap-
frozen by dimethylbutane pre-cooled at freezing point and
subsequently immersed in liquid nitrogen. All tissues listed
in the Tables were sectioned and parts of all, except the
hippocampus, cardiac lobes and diaphragmatic lobes, were used
for virus isolation.

Cell cultures and virus isolation

Primary cultures of pig kidney (PK_1) cells were prepared
from healthy three to five week old piglets from the Institute's

* MK-25, Pharmachim, Sofia, Bulgaria and Ayvac, Pliva, Zagreb, Yugoslavia.

farm. Secondary monolayers of PK cells were grown in milk
dilution bottles (Kimax) and disposable petri dishes* (ϕ 6.0 cm)
at $37^{\circ}C$ in a humidified CO_2 incubator. Growth medium consisted
of Earle's BSS, supplemented with 0.002% phenol red, amino
acids and vitamins (Eagle, 1955) and 10% lamb serum. Penicillin,
streptomycin and mycostatin were incorporated at 200 units/ml,
0.2 mg/ml and 100 units/ml respectively. The same medium
(Earle-MEM), but with 2% lamb serum was used as maintenance
medium.

Tissue extracts (4 - 10% w/v dependent on the amount
available), were prepared in maintenance medium by grinding
and centrifugation at 2 000 r.p.m. for 10 min. The medium used
for tissue extracts contained twice the normal amounts of
penicillin, streptomycin, mycostatin and 30 units/ml polymixin
B and 0.2 mg/ml kanamycin.

The PK_2 cell monolayer of a milk dilution bottle was
inoculated with 2 - 4 ml tissue extract for the purpose of
virus isolation. After adsorption for 1 h at $37^{\circ}C$, the inoculum
was replaced by maintenance medium. Cultures were examined
microscopically for CPE for up to seven days. In case of doubt
a sub-inoculation was made. Isolates were identified as ADV
by means of plaque neutralisation, using a monospecific hyperimmune serum.

For quantitative virus studies two petri dishes with PK_2
cell monolayers were each inoculated with 0.5 ml tissue
extract. After adsorption, the monolayers were overlayed with
1% methyl cellulose in maintenance medium. The cultures were
incubated for a further 4 - 6 days and then stained with amido
black.

Detection of antigen

Cryostat sections of tissues from vaccinated and control
piglets were stained with a swine anti-AD-virus γ globulin,
conjugated with fluorescein-isothiocyanate. The conjugate was
kindly provided by Dr. R.M.S. Wirahadiredja, Central Veterinary
Institute, Rotterdam and was the same as that used in regional

* Falcon

veterinary laboratories. The sections were examined for
fluorescence with a Leitz Ortholux microscope fitted with a
dark field condenser and illuminated by an Osram (HBO-200)
lamp.

Histopathology

Cryostat sections of frozen tissues were stained with
haematoxylin and eosin and examined by ordinary light micro-
scopy for the presence of perivascular and focal lesions.

RESULTS

Piglets vaccinated with strain MK-25 and strain Ayvak
received $10^{4.4}$ and $10^{3.1}$ p.f.u. respectively, whereas the
control pigs were inoculated with $10^{5.0}$ p.f.u. of strain NIA-3.
Fluorescence could not be observed in any tissue sample of the
eight piglets autopsied at 4, 7, 10 and 14 days after vaccination with strain MK-25. Also ADV could not be isolated and
no histopathologic lesions were found. On the other hand, virus
was recovered from both piglets killed four days after vaccination with the Ayvak strain. All parts of the brain of pig
no. 1, except the cortex, and the lung of pig no. 2 yielded
virus (Table 1).

Immunofluorescence and histopathology, however, failed
to show the presence of an ADV infection in the two piglets.
The other six piglets of this litter were found negative by all
methods.

The control piglets inoculated with strain NIA-3 showed a
rise in body temperature, anorexia and dullness on the following days. Pig no. 9 lost control of balance and was found dead
on the fourth day post inoculation, when no. 10 was killed.
Virus was recovered from all tissues of the piglet that died
and from all but one of the animal that was killed (Table 2).
In piglet no. 9 fluorescence was observed in one of the cardiac
lobes only, whereas a single isolated lesion of perivascular
cuffing was seen in the thalamus. On the other hand, no
fluorescence was detected in the tissues of the piglet that
 as killed, although perivascular cuffing and foci of mono-
 uclear cells were found in all parts of the brain.

TABLE 1

DIAGNOSTIC RESULTS FOUR DAYS AFTER VACCINATION WITH STRAIN AYVAK

Tissue	Pig no. 1			Pig no. 2		
	IFT	$\log_{10}$ p.f.u./g	Histo-path.	IFT	$\log_{10}$ p.f.u./g	Histo-path.
Cerebral cortex	−	−	−	−	−	−
Hippocampus	−	NT	−	−	NT	−
Thalamus	−	1.0	−	−	−	−
Cerebellum	−	1.0	−	−	−	−
Trigeminal area	−	+[1]	−	−	−	−
Pons	−	1.4	−	−	−	−
Medulla oblongata	−	+	−	−	−	−
Tonsils	−	−	−	−	−	−
Apical lobes	−	−	−	−	1.8	−
Cardiac lobes	−	NT	−	−	NT	−
Diaphragmatic lobes	−	NT	−	−	NT	−

[1] Virus recovered in bottle cultures only

TABLE 2

DIAGNOSTIC RESULTS FOUR DAYS AFTER INTRAMUSCULAR INOCULATION OF STRAIN NIA-3 VIRUS

Tissue	Pig no. 9 (died)			Pig no. 10 (killed)		
	IFT	$\log_{10}$ p.f.u./g	Histo-path.	IFT	$\log_{10}$ p.f.u./g	Histo-path.
Cerebral cortex	−	1.6	−	−	2.1	+
Hippocampus	−	NT	−	−	NT	+
Thalamus	−	2.9	+	−	1.6	+
Cerebellum	−	2.8	−	−	1.8	+
Trigeminal area	−	3.4	−	−	+[1]	+
Pons	−	3.5	−	−	−	+
Medulla oblongata	−	4.1	−	−	2.0	+
Tonsils	−	4.7	−	−	3.7	−
Apical lobes	−	2.9	−	−	2.5	−
Cardiac lobes	+	NT	−	−	NT	−
Diaphragmatic lobes	−	NT	−	−	NT	−

[1] Virus recovered in bottle cultures only

DISCUSSION

Laboratory diagnosis of AD is usually based on virus isolation from brain and tonsils (Akkermans, 1963), detection of viral antigen by immunofluorescence in brain, tonsils and lungs (Meyling and Bitsch, 1967; Sabó and Rajcáni, 1969) or on histopathological lesions of the brain (Fankhauser and Wyler, 1953; Done et al., 1957). Our results indicate that vaccination with MLV vaccines is not likely to interfere with the laboratory diagnosis of AD field strains. The Ayvak vaccine, however, can cause a false positive diagnosis, if virus isolation is employed.

The question arises whether the almost complete absence of ADV and the absence of histopathological lesions following vaccination should be attributed solely to the properties of the two MLV strains or perhaps also to the route of inoculation. The virus titres of tissues after intramuscular inoculation with NIA-3 virus were substantially higher than those observed after intramuscular vaccination with Ayvak virus (Tables 1 and 2), and nearly reached the level which is seen after intranasal application of NIA-3 virus (De Leeuw, personal communication). The aspects and distribution of histopathological lesions in the central nervous system of one of the control piglets (Table 2) were in accordance with the changes described by Fankhauser and Wyler (1953). It seems, therefore, that the general lack of virus and histopathological lesions after vaccination should be ascribed to the properties of the vaccine viruses, rather than to the route of application. The central nervous lesions of the two control pigs, however, were inconsistent with the severity of the clinical signs, the course of disease and virus titres. Although the reason for the discrepancy remains obscure, it questions the reliability of histopathological methods as a diagnostic tool for AD.

Taking into account the age at which pigs in the field are usually vaccinated for the first time, it appears highly unlikely that AD would be diagnosed as a result of vaccination with the MLV vaccines studied, if histopathologic or immunofluorescent methods are used.

ACKNOWLEDGEMENTS

The authors are indebted to Dr. P.W. de Leeuw and Dr. J.Th. van Oirschot for valuable suggestions in designing the experiment. The skilful technical assistance of Messrs. F.E. van Alphen and H.C. van Mourik is gratefully appreciated.

REFERENCES

Akkermans, J.P.W.M. 1963. Ziekte van Aujeszky bij het varken in Nederland. Thesis, University Utrecht, 43-45.
Done, J.T. 1957. The pathological differentiation of diseases of the central nervous system. Vet. Rec., 69, 1341-1349.
Eagle, H. 1955. Nutrition needs of mammalian cells in tissue culture. Science, 122, 501-504.
Fankhauser, R. and Wyler, R. 1953. Die Nervenkrankheiten des Schweines. Schw. Arch. Tierh., 95, 585-619.
De Leeuw, P.W. and Tiessink, J.W.A. 1980. Recent studies on Aujeszky's Disease in Pigs and Cattle. Tijdschr. Diergeneesk., 105, 689-694.
Meyling, A. and Bitsch, V. 1967. The diagnosis of pseudorabies by the fluorescent antibody technique. Acta Vet. Scand., 8, 360-368.
Sabó, A. and Rajcáni, J. 1970. Rapid diagnosis of Aujeszky's disease by the fluorescent antibody technique. Acta virol. Prague, 14, 475-484.

SEROLOGICAL DIAGNOSIS OF AUJESZKY'S DISEASE USING ENZYME-LINKED IMMUNOSORBENT ASSAY (ELISA)

B. Toma

Chaire des Maladies Contagieuses
Ecole Nationale Vétérinaire d'Alfort
F-94704 Maisons-Alfort Cedex, France.

ABSTRACT

The ELISA has been developed for the detection of Aujeszky's disease virus (ADV) antibodies. Several hundred sera have been studied comparatively using the ELISA and seroneutralisation techniques. The results obtained by the two techniques were very similar. The advantages of ELISA make it ideal for epidemiological surveys and the large scale, early detection of antibodies to ADV.

INTRODUCTION

The ELISA has numerous advantages that have led many research teams to apply it for the early detection of antibodies or the diagnosis of diverse human or animal diseases.

For Aujeszky's disease (AD), the first results were published in 1978 (Moutou et al., 1978). Other teams then published their results (Briaire et al., 1979; Bommeli et al., 1980). Now, several laboratories use the ELISA for Aujeszky's disease virus (ADV) antibody testing, even though their results have not yet been published (Toma, 1981).

At the Contagious Diseases Laboratory of the National Veterinary School at Alfort, an indirect method was developed using a pig globulin antiserum labelled by an enzyme (Toma et al., 1979). This technique was then modified and the anti-pig globulin antiserum was replaced by anti-pig IgA antiserum labelled by an enzyme.

The following text gives the details of the latter technique and the results obtained during a comparative study of pig sera using the ELISA and seroneutralisation.

G. Wittmann, S.A. Hall (eds), Aujeszky's Disease. ISBN-13:978-94-009-7555-2

MATERIALS AND METHODS

1)   MATERIALS

Antigens

     A layer of TFP cells in serum-free MEM pyruvate medium
was infected by an ADV strain. After 24 hours, the cells were
unstuck by the joint action of a 4°/oo KCl solution and carefully shaken glass beads. The cell suspension was then centrifuged at 700 g for 10 minutes in an oblique rotor and the
sediment washed three times in a KCl solution. The last sediment was resuspended in KCl Triton X 100 (2°/oo) and the cell
debris enucleated in Dounce's potter. The mixture was then
passed on KCl sucrose (0.25M) for 10 minutes at 700 g. The
sediment was resuspended in Tris EDTA (pH 9.6) in 1/50th of
the volume of the initial culture medium; this antigen was
stored at -70^oC.

     A control antigen was prepared in exactly the same way,
apart from the inoculation of the virus.

Sera

     Various groups of sera were obtained as follows:

a)   15 pigs were used to provide sera for studies on antibody
      kinetics:
            3 controls
            3 inoculated once with Alfort 26 strain, then
            virulent challenge
            3 inoculated twice with Alfort 26 strain, then
            virulent challenge
            1 inoculated once with Alfort 26 strain
            5 inoculated twice with Alfort 26 strain.

b)   487 serum samples from sows and meat pigs were collected
      from 46 herds which were either free from AD, infected
      or vaccinated;

c)   30 American serum samples.

Apparatus

Multiwash (Dynatech)

Multiskan (Dynatech)

Reagents and plates

a) Serum diluent
PBS Tween 20 solution 0.05%:
PBS (10 x conc) . . . . . 100 ml
de-ionised water . . 900 ml pH 7.2
+ 0.05 ml of Tween 20 (polyoxyethylene sorbitane mono laureate) (Merck)

b) Diluent for the IgA - peroxidase conjugate
PBS Tween 20 solution 0.05% - Bovine albumin 1%:
Bovine albumin fraction V Sigma.

c) Substrate:
Orthophenylene diamine . . . . 4 mg
in citrate phosphate buffer pH 5.0 . . . 10 ml
H_2O_2 10 v . . . . 0.15 ml

d) Citrate phosphate buffer solution pH 5.0
citric acid 0.1 M . . . . 243 ml
disodium phosphate 0.2 M . . . . 257 ml
de-ionised water . . . . .1 000 ml

e) M 129 B plates

2) METHODS

ELISA

The wells of the plates were sensitised with 200 µl of a viral antigen suspension for columns No. 1, 3, 5, 7 and 11 and with a control antigen suspension for columns 2, 4, 6, 8, 10 and 12.

The plate was placed on an antistatic cushion and 200 µl of 1/30th diluted sera in PBS Tween 20 at 0.05% were put in the wells. The sera were diluted in small rhesus tubes, then redistributed with a multi-canal pipette with a disposable tip.

For each serum there was a control well and a well containing viral antigen. On each plate there was also a negative reference serum and a positive reference serum.

The plate was covered by a plastic cover and incubated for 1/2 hour at $37^{\circ}C$ on a slow balancing stirrer. It was then rinsed with the Multiwash apparatus (2 times plot 3): distilled water/Tween 20 at 0.05%.

The IgA-peroxidase was resuspended with 1 ml of distilled water and then diluted in 79 ml of PBS-Tween 20 containing 1% bovine albumin. This amount of reagent was enough for 4 plates; 200 µl of the conjugate solution were put into each well. After incubation for one hour at + $37^{\circ}C$ on a slow balancing stirrer, the plate was rinsed with the Multiwash apparatus (2 times plot 3) with distilled water + Tween 20 at 0.05%.

The tracer mixture of the enzyme was prepared and then put into the wells at a rate of 200 µl per well, protected from all light sources. The plates were kept for 15 minutes at laboratory temperature and protected from light. At the end of this period, the reaction was stopped by adding 50 µl of 2N sulphuric acid to each well.

The results were read with the Multiskan apparatus with 510 nm wavelength. The zero calibration of the machine was made on an empty plate.

Expression of the results

The optical density (OD) of the serum in the presence of the control cell antigen was subtracted from the OD of the same serum in the presence of the viral antigen. The figure obtained was multiplied by 10. Only one figure was kept after the decimal point.

    Example: OD serum with control cell antigen: 0.346
               OD serum with viral antigen: 1.259
                      1.259 - 0.346 =   0.913
                              Index   =   9.1

Interpretation of the results

From a study of several hundred sera with titres determined by seroneutralisation, the following criteria were adopted for the interpretation of the results of the ELISA:

ELISA index less than 1 - negative

ELISA index more than 1 but less than 2 - the specimen is retested. If the index is then higher than 1 it is considered positive

ELISA index more than 2 - positive

Seroneutralisation test

The technique for this has already been published (Toma and Vannier, 1980).

RESULTS

Antibody kinetics study

Examples of kinetics are given in Figures 1 and 2. Generally speaking, the development of the antibody titres measured by the two techniques was almost parallel. After being in contact with the ADV, the response of animals became positive with the ELISA technique at the same time or earlier than with seroneutralisation.

Field sera study

The results have been presented by distinguishing on the one hand pig farms free from ADV, and on the other hand, pig farms where the animals have been vaccinated or infected by the ADV.

a)   Pig farms free of ADV

Two hundred and sixty five samples of sera from sows or meat pigs from 23 pig farms free of the disease were submitted to the two techniques. All these sera gave a negative response with seroneutralisation. The responses were also negative with the ELISA technique. The distribution of the ELISA indices obtained with these 265 serum samples is shown in Figure 3.

b)   Pig farms with vaccinated or infected animals

Serum samples of 222 sows and meat pigs from 23 pig farms were studied. Results are shown in Table 1.

70

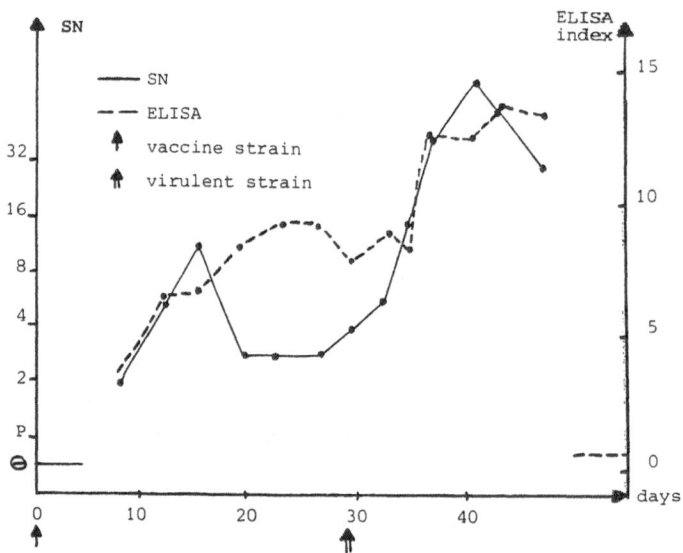

Fig. 1.   Comparative development of antibodies revealed by seroneutralisation
or by the ELISA in the serum of a pig injected once with the Alfort
26 strain, and then challenged with a virulent strain.

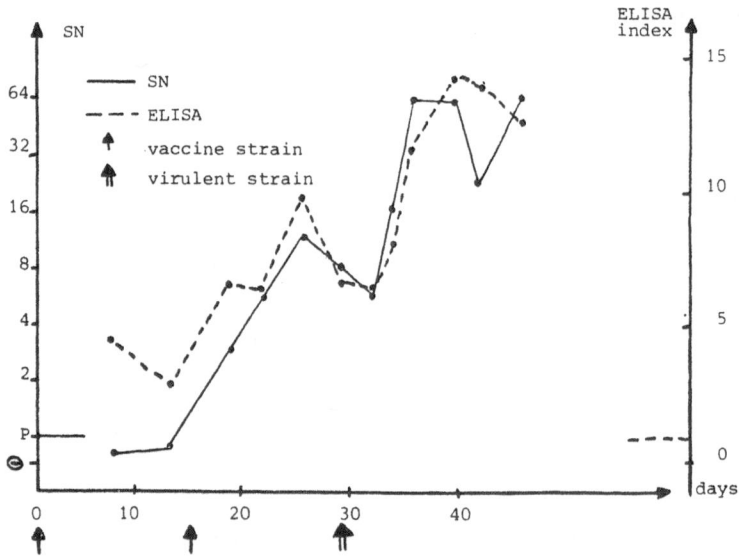

Fig. 2.   Comparative development of antibodies revealed by seroneutralisation
or by the ELISA in the serum of a pig injected twice with the Alfort
26 strain, and then challenged with a virulent strain.

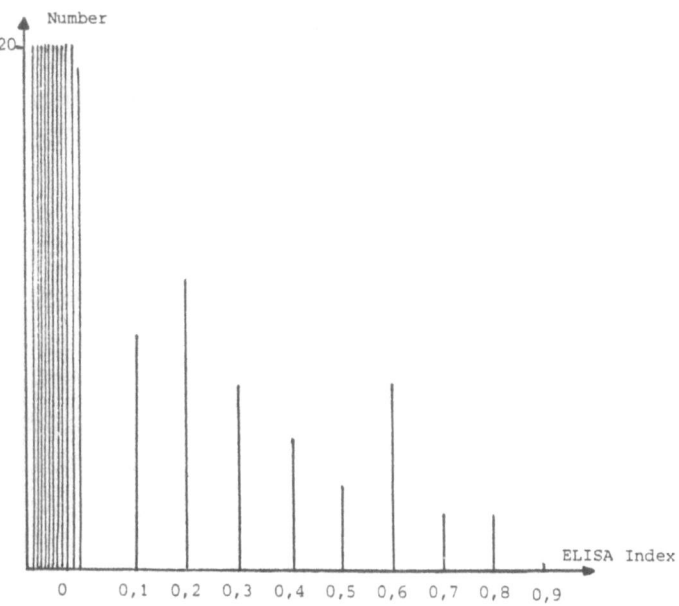

Fig. 3.   Histogram illustrating the distribution of the ELISA indices for
          the 265 serum samples from pig farms free from ADV.

TABLE 1

COMPARISON OF RESULTS OBTAINED WITH THE ELISA TECHNIQUE AND SERO-
NEUTRALISATION OF 222 SERUM SAMPLES FROM INFECTED OR VACCINATED PIG FARMS

Seroneutralisation	ELISA	
Positive response : 127	Positive response :	127
Doubtful response : 1	Positive response :	1
Negative response : 86	Positive response :	2
	Negative response :	84
Cytotoxic sera : 8	Positive response :	6
	Negative response :	2

All the sera found to be positive in the seroneutralisation test gave a positive response with the ELISA.
The ELISA response enabled two serum samples, probably possessing a low amount of AD viral antibody (index numbers 1.8 and
2.2), to be noted and, for the 8 serum samples that had a
cytotoxic action hindering the seroneutralisation test, the
ELISA provided a result.

For the 127 serum samples that gave a positive seroneutralisation test result, a histogram of the ELISA index
distribution is shown in Figure 4.

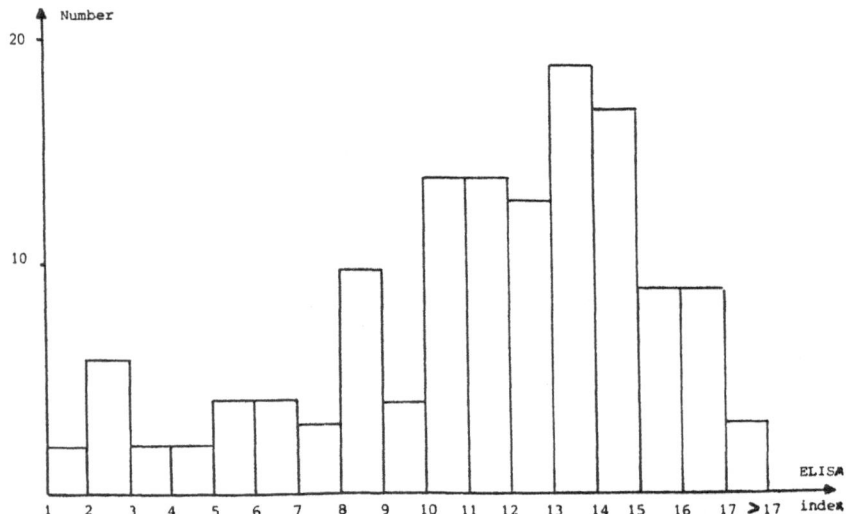

Fig. 4. Histogram illustrating the distribution of the ELISA indices
for the 127 serum samples which gave a positive response in
seroneutralisation.

The ELISA and seroneutralisation test results in this
comparative study of the sera of sows and of meat pigs, either
vaccinated or infected, were very similar. The sera of piglets
born of vaccinated sows were also studied. The differences
were more numerous due to the low level of antibodies of
colostral origin being below the limit of sensitivity of one
or other of the techniques.

Comparative titration of serum tests

The 30 American test sera were submitted to seroneutralisation and ELISA at Alfort.   Results obtained can be
seen in Figure 5.   An excellent correlation between the titres
obtained with both techniques can be noted.

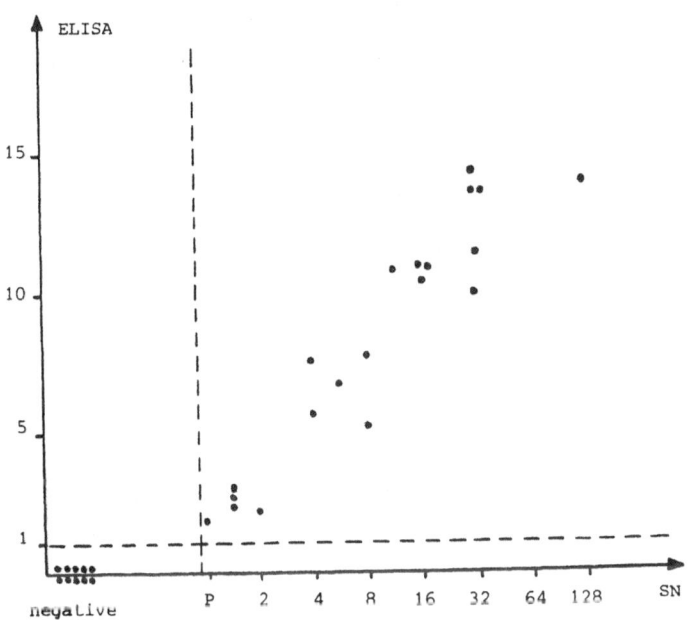

Fig. 5.   Correlation between the titres obtained by seroneutralisation or by
the ELISA on the 30 American test sera.

DISCUSSION

The ELISA technique that has been developed possesses a
sensitivity near to that of the seroneutralisation technique
used at Alfort and this could probably be improved even further
to reach that obtained by other research teams.   However, the
ELISA is now used routinely for the diagnosis of AD and early
detection of AD viral antibody.   Its advantages are undeniable:
limited cost, early responses, partly automatable and quantitative result with a single dilution.   It can readily be used

for epidemiological surveys and large scale early detection of
disease.

It now remains to complete a comparative study of the
ELISA techniques developed by various teams so that the best
cost-effective method can be selected.

ACKNOWLEDGEMENT

The author thanks Martine Pezron and Micheline Bailly for
their technical assistance.

REFERENCES

Briaire, J., Meloen, R.H. and Barteling, S.J., 1979. An enzyme-linked
    immunosorbent assay (ELISA) for the detection of antibody against
    Aujeszky's disease virus in pig sera. Zbl. Vet. Med. B, 26, 76-81.
Bommeli, W.R., Kihm, U., Lazarowicz, M. and Steck, F., 1980. Rapid
    detection of antibodies to infectious bovine rhinotracheitis (IBR)
    virus by micro enzyme linked immunosorbent assay (micro-ELISA). 2nd
    International Symposium of Veterinary Laboratory Diagnosticians, 2,
    235-239.
Moutou, F., Toma, B. and Fortier, B., 1978. Application of an enzyme linked
    immunosorbent assay (ELISA) for diagnosis of Aujeszky's disease in
    swine. Vet. Rec., 103, 264.
Toma, B., Moutou, F. and Fortier, B., 1979. Recherche des anticorps anti-
    virus de la maladie d'Aujeszky par la technique ELISA. Rec. Méd.
    Vét., 155 (5), 455-463.
Toma, B. and Vannier, P., 1980. Harmonization attempt between French
    laboratories involved in the research of neutralizing antibodies
    against pseudorabies virus or transmissible gastroenteritis virus.
    2nd International Symposium of Veterinary Laboratory Diagnosticians,
    Lucerne, Paper 1.
Toma, B., 1981. Harmonisation between European laboratories regarding the
    seroneutralisation of Aujeszky's disease virus. Proc. CEC Seminar
    on Aujeszky's disease, Tübingen, June, 1981 (this publication).

HARMONISATION BETWEEN EUROPEAN LABORATORIES ON THE SERONEUTRALISATION TEST FOR AUJESZKY'S DISEASE VIRUS

B. Toma

Chaire des Maladies Contagieuses
Ecole Nationale Vétérinaire d'Alfort,
F-94704 Maisons-Alfort Cedex, France.

ABSTRACT

Two preliminary series of blind studies of serum samples in French laboratories practising serological diagnosis of Aujeszky's disease (AD) by seroneutralisation, led to the recommendation of a technical protocol for this test and to the determination of a reference serum corresponding to a possible grade of sensitivity. A third series of studies made jointly with some European laboratories established the average sensitivity of the techniques used by these laboratories and the concentration of antibodies that could be adopted for an international reference serum. Further complementary studies are envisaged, especially with American laboratories, so that harmonisation in Aujeszky's disease virus (ADV) antibody titration may be achieved.

INTRODUCTION

Over the past few years the increasing incidence of Aujeszky's disease (AD) in several countries (Western Europe, USA, Singapore, etc.) has led to the introduction of regulations for its diagnosis and control. It seems certain that this trend will lead to the adoption of import controls and the testing of pigs in the course of international trade.

Research into the vaccination of pigs against AD has progressed in recent years and some results have already been published. However, owing to differences in the serological techniques used to evaluate the humoral immune response and a lack of standard reference sera, it is difficult to compare results obtained by different research teams.

It thus seemed necessary to begin a study with the aim of harmonising the serological results obtained in different countries and adopting an international reference serum. The use of a reference serum is the only way that research teams can communicate internationally on the same wavelength regarding serological tests and it is the only way that will allow

G. Wittmann, S.A. Hall (eds), Aujeszky's Disease. ISBN-13:978-94-009-7555-2

comparison of the humoral immunity conferred by vaccines studied in different countries.

The first phase of this study was done in France, with a view to harmonising techniques and results in those French laboratories practising AD serological diagnosis. It consisted of a blind study of various sera and it showed significant differences in the results obtained by the different laboratories. The second phase, in which some other European laboratories were included, led to the proposal of technical guidelines for seroneutralisation tests combining convenience, specificity and sensitivity. It also led to the definition of the concentration of neutralising antibodies that constituted a positive threshold for the seroneutralisation test and a definition for the reference serum adopted by the French laboratories.

The third phase was a study of a new series of sera by French laboratories and some European laboratories. In the following paragraphs, we intend only to relate results obtained during the third phase, as earlier results have already been reported (Toma and Vannier, 1980).

MATERIALS AND METHODS

The study concerned 30 samples corresponding to dilutions of two positive, and two negative sera.

The first positive serum (No. 1) included two samples for each of six dilutions ranging from 1/180 to 1/5 960 (common difference 2). It was a porcine, SPF, ADV hyperimmune serum whose 1/180 dilution was proposed as the positive threshold in French laboratories at the end of phase 2.

The second positive serum (No. 2) corresponded to 16 samples distributed in 9 dilutions ranging from 1/100 to 1/50 000. It was a porcine, ADV hyperimmune serum, available on the market, which was already used as a comparison for the results over time.

Twenty laboratories studied these 30 sera: 11 French laboratories* and 9 European laboratories**.

The seroneutralisation tests used by the laboratories differed considerably in technical details: number of $CCID_{50}$ of AD virus, virus/serum incubation time, volume of reagent used etc.

RESULTS

Nine out of eleven French laboratories obtained concordant results in this study; the percentage of positive or doubtful results varied from 32% to 65%.

For the European laboratories, the percentage of positive or doubtful results varied from 21% to 86%.

Figures 1 to 4 demonstrate results obtained by French and European laboratories in direct relation with the dilution of positive sera.

Some laboratories studied the 30 samples with both the seroneutralisation test and the ELISA. Their results are shown in Table 1.

TABLE 1

COMPARISON OF RESULTS OBTAINED BY 4 LABORATORIES WITH THE ELISA AND SERO-NEUTRALISATION

| | Percentage of positive or doubtful results | | | |
	Lab. 1	Lab. 2	Lab. 3	Lab. 4
Seroneutralisation	46	32	57	21
ELISA	39	46	79	59

* Chappuis (Lyon), Duée (Lille), Gayot and Ursache (Alfort), Goffaux (Alfort), Goyon (Le Mans), Guerche (Tours), Lorant (St. Brieuc), Renault (Athis-Mons), Szymanski (Château-Thierry), Toma (Alfort) and Vannier (Ploufragan).

** Bommeli (Switzerland), Borst (Holland), Cartwright (GB), Kabelik (Czechoslovakia), Leunen and Biront (Belgium), McNulty (N. Ireland), Moscari (Hungary), Pensaert (Belgium) and Rondhuis (Holland).

78

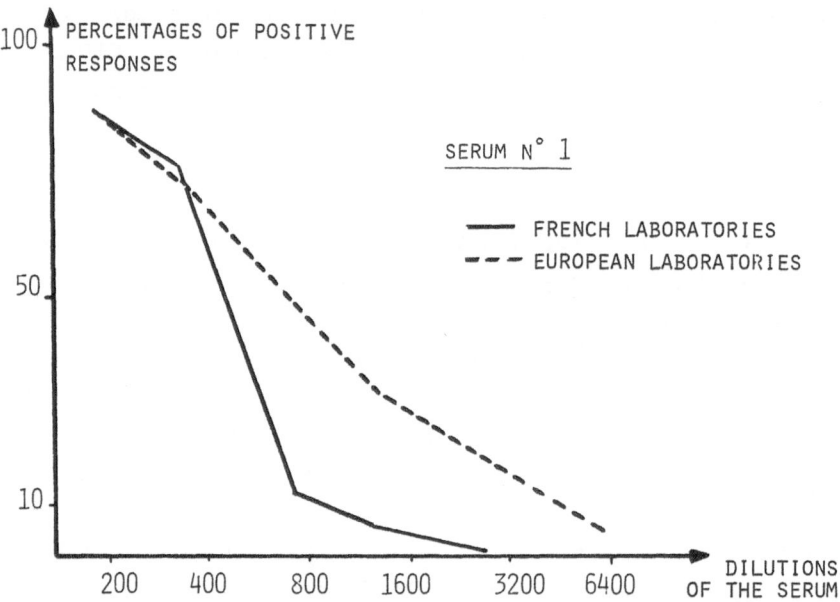

Fig. 1. Percentage of definitely positive results óbtained by French or
other European laboratories with dilutions of positive serum No. 1.

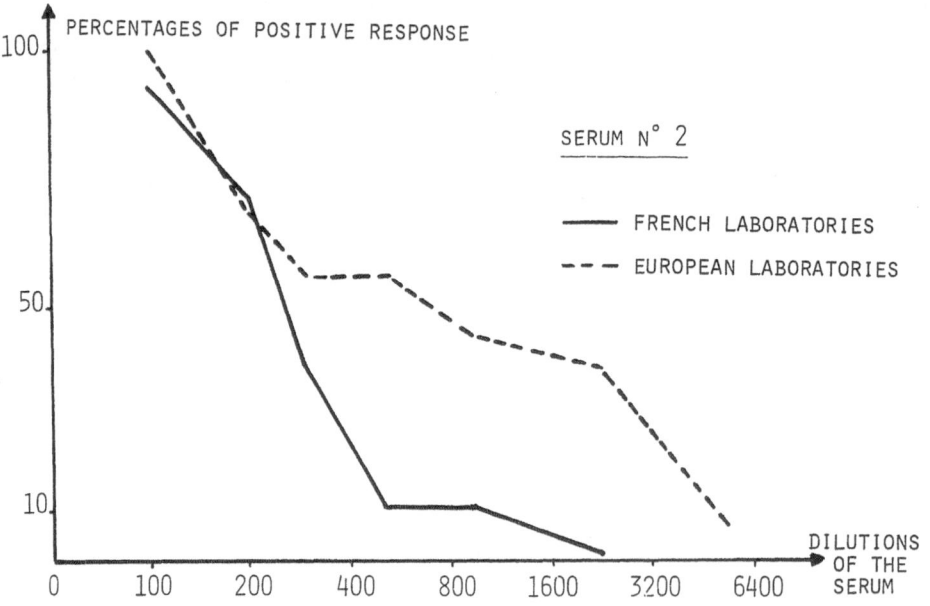

Fig. ?. Percentage of definitely positive results obtained by French or
other European laboratories with dilutions of positive serum No. 2.

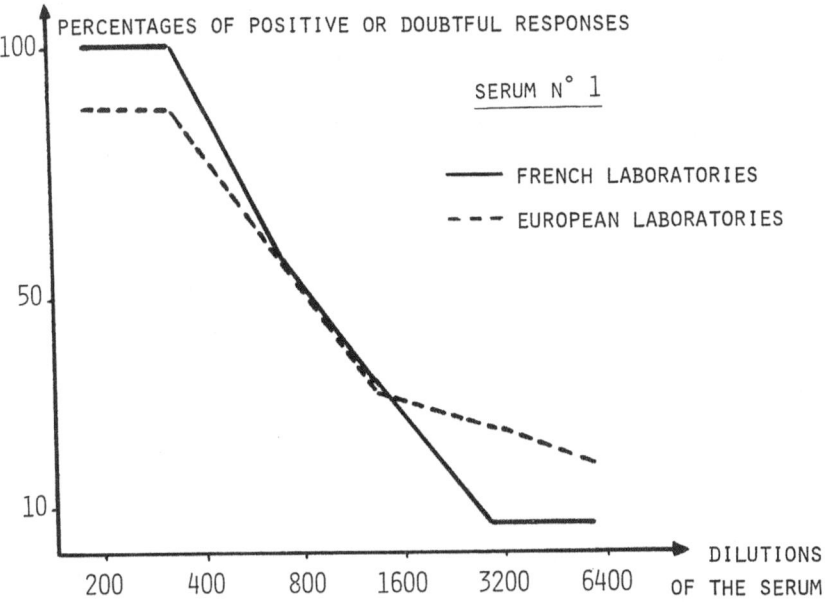

Fig. 3.   Percentage of positive or doubtful responses obtained by French or
other European laboratories with positive serum No. 1.

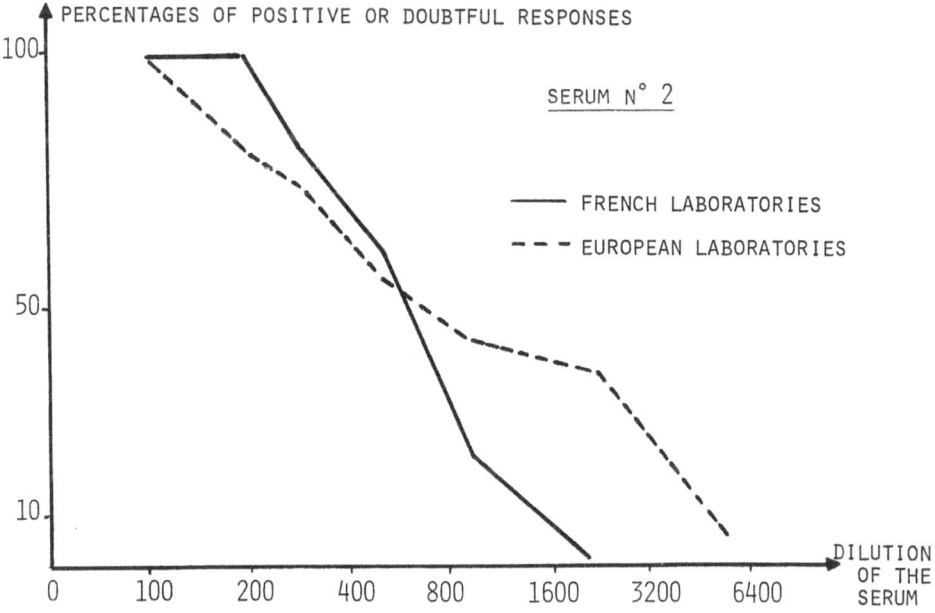

Fig. 4.   Percentage of positive or doubtful responses obtained by French or
other European laboratories with positive serum No. 2.

The French Reference Serum was studied by different European laboratories both as the reference serum and blindly, in a 1/180 dilution of positive serum No. 1. The titres varied between 2 and 8 with one exception: one laboratory had a negative result with this serum.

A French laboratory made a study on the reference serum by varying the number of $CCID_{50}$ of the virus. Results are given in Table 2.

TABLE 2

RESULTS OBTAINED BY ONE LABORATORY WITH THE FRENCH REFERENCE SERUM (MICRO-PLATES, VIRUS/SERUM CONTACT TIME: 1 h AT 37°C)

| | Number of $CCID_{50}$ | | | | |
	10	50	100	500	1 000
Pure reference serum	0/14*	0/14	0/14	2/14	14/14
1/2 diluted reference serum	0/14	3/14	5/14	12/14	14/14
1/4 diluted reference serum	4/14	8/14	14/14	14/14	14/14

* Number of wells with CPE/number of wells used.

The results illustrate the differences obtained in relation to the number of $CCID_{50}$ of virus used. Similar results could be obtained by varying the virus/serum contact time.

DISCUSSION

The study of Figures 1 to 4 shows that the percentage of definitely positive results was higher for European laboratories than for French laboratories; there was less difference between them when definitely positive results and doubtful results were compared.

These results show that 56% of French or European laboratories obtained a positive or doubtful response with positive serum No. 1 diluted to 1/720 (which corresponds to the reference serum diluted to 1/4).

The ELISA generally proved to be more sensitive than seroneutralisation (Table 1).

Taking into account the results of the different laboratories and the necessity for keeping the test simple and easy to use, we propose the following:

French freeze-dried reference serum reconstituted in 1 ml of distilled water (which corresponds to positive serum No. 1 diluted to 1/180): should be found positive in 100% of all tests;

French freeze-dried reference serum reconstituted in 2 ml of distilled water (corresponding to positive serum No. 1 diluted to 1/360): should be found positive or doubtful;

French freeze-dried reference serum reconstituted in 4 ml of distilled water (corresponding to positive serum No. 1 diluted to 1/720): negative or doubtful.

These proposals and this serum should be submitted to more European laboratories who regularly practise AD diagnosis by seroneutralisation or by other methods.

It is obvious that there will continue to be differences in the accuracy of the techniques used by the laboratories, depending on the number of $CCID_{50}$, the virus/serum contact time and the temperature. However, it seems highly desirable to adopt an international reference reagent, of an antibody level sufficient for detection by all laboratories so that it may be used to make comparisons and express results in standard ADV antibody titres.

A study is under way with the National Animal Disease Centre , Ames, Iowa, which, two years ago made a similar study in the States on inter-laboratory differences in ADV serology test results (Stewart et al., 1980).

Comparison of the European results with the American results should enable an international ADV reference serum to be defined.

ACKNOWLEDGEMENT

The author thanks Martine Pezron and Micheline Bailly for their technical assistance.

82

REFERENCES

Stewart, W.C., Swanson, M.R. and Eernisse, K.A., 1980. A program to
        monitor and improve the proficiency of laboratories performing the
        neutralisation test for pseudorabies. Proc. Int. Pig. Vet. Soc.
        Congress, Copenhagen, p. 102.
Toma, B. and Vannier, P., 1980. Harmonization attempt between French
        laboratories involved in the research of neutralizing antibodies
        against pseudorabies virus or transmissible gastroenteritis virus,
        2nd. Int. Symp. Vet. Lab. Diagn., Lucerne, 1-4.

GENERAL DISCUSSION

B. Toma *(France)* I suggest we divide this general discussion period into separate topics. The first could be seroneutralis- ation in relation to Dr. Bitsch's paper. The second topic could be the ELISA. A third topic could be the harmonisation of techniques and results between laboratories.

R.J. Lorenz *(Federal Republic of Germany)* Dr. Bitsch, did you also consider that the kinetics of seroneutralisation could be reversible? I remember that in the early models that were made on the neutralisation process, the people concerned con- sidered that this process might not be irreversible.

V. Bitsch *(Denmark)* I have considered that possibility. We published on that in 1978. We explained this seroneutralis- ation phenomenon partly by the fact that we had virus antibody combinations, between virus-antibody complexes, that were non- infectious but which would be dissociated on dilution. The straight lines would then be explained by non-soluble virus- antibody complexes. We have also tried to dissociate the virus-antibody complexes by dilution and after short pre- incubations we were able to provoke dissociation between virus and antibody. After longer pre-incubation periods it was almost impossible. Therefore, we concluded that the virus antibody combinations produced late in the course of the neutralisation test were mainly non-soluble virus-antibody complexes.

R.J. Lorenz Thank you. Now I have a question for Dr. Moennig. You presented a very good four-fold table comparing the positive and negative results in the ELISA and in the serum neutralis- ation test. There were six discordant results which were positive in the ELISA and negative in the serum neutralisation test. Could that mean that the ELISA technique is less specific than the neutralisation test?

V. Moennig *(Federal Republic of Germany)* I should have mentioned that all these discrepancies were in the very low titre region. That is, we observed discrepancies with the neutralisation test in a serum dilution of 1 in 2, and we observed the discrepancies

with the ELISA only with 1 in 20. So, I cannot answer your
question exactly. It may be that the ELISA is not as specific
as one would wish in low dilutions. However, it could also
mean that it detects very low amounts of serum antibodies
earlier. I am not in a position to say yes or no to this
question, but one has to think of these two possibilities. In
principle you are right, with the ELISA you have an optical
density which you either believe or disbelieve, whereas with
the serum neutralisation test you have a specific activity
which neutralises the serum. I think at present that it is
too early to give a definite explanation of the phenomenon.

R.J. Lorenz   I have heard recently from a number of people
who hold the opinion that the ELISA is much more sensitive than
the neutralisation technique but that it has a serious disadvantage in being less specific. Would you agree?

V. Moennig   I will disagree if we are talking about the ELISA
in general terms. It depends very much on the reagents you
use. In our laboratory I have to admit that our first ELISAs
had a very low specificity. However, you can do a lot of things
to improve specificity and the fact that you have the control
wells with a negative antigen gives you much more security
with regard to specificity. So I think that the opinion that
the ELISA is less specific than the neutralisation test is
largely dependent on the question of the quality of the reagent.
The reagent we used came from Behringwerke in Marburg and
seemed to be very specific, with the one exception of the low
titre region. For this we thought of starting serum dilutions
with 1 in 40 to avoid the problems.

B. Toma   When someone says he has six positive sera, or six
negative sera, in the serum neutralisation test, it depends
totally on the technique that is used. I don't know exactly
what your technique is but I am sure that if you gave to Dr.
Bitsch your six negative serum neutralisation sera which are
positive by ELISA, he would find them to be strongly positive.

V. Moennig   I must point out that, as I said, we do not add
complement to our tests. We just use a standard neutralisation

test which is probably less sensitive than other tests that are being used.

B. Toma   I am just making the point that your test has a one hour incubation time, at 37°C, without complement. If you compare that with Dr. Bitsch's technique, that is 24 hours, with complement, you have perhaps a factor of 20 between the results, between the titres.

V. Bitsch   I would like to ask Dr. Moennig and Dr. Toma, why they are so reluctant to accept a neutralisation test with a longer pre-incubation period at 37°C. Dr. Moennig: you used a neutralisation test with conventional pre-incubation conditions and you tested serum diluted 1 in 2. If you had tested serum undiluted you would probably have found that the ELISA positives were also positive in the neutralisation test. One other thing, if you don't want to use the full sensitivity of a test with a pre-incubation at 37°C for 24 hours, you could test serum diluted 1 in 4 or 1 in 8, instead of 1 in 2 or undiluted. Then you would save serum.

V. Moennig   I have to admit that we were fairly careless about the performance of the serum neutralisation test but our object was to use exactly the serum neutralisation test which is most commonly used. We though that the addition of complement might complicate the test, especially where it is necessary to screen large numbers of sera.   So we used a very simple test, always keeping in mind the application to screening large numbers of sera. If you add complement you run into another problem; you have to titrate your complement every time you use it; you have to have a standardised complement system, and all this makes the whole thing more complicated.

V. Bitsch   Yes, but I think you have misunderstood something because our standard neutralisation test is not a test with the incorporation of complement. In certain cases there are advantages in incorporating complement in a neutralisation test but it is not a test that would be necessary in routine examinations. Our conventional test, without the addition of complement, is sensitive enough to detect all antibody carriers. That is our conclusion at least.

<u>B. Toma</u>   I think that this discussion shows the necessity of having a common reference serum to enable us to make exact comparisons between laboratories.

<u>H. Ludwig</u>   *(Federal Republic of Germany)*   I think one must differentiate clearly between the various purposes for which the ELISA is used; between using the ELISA for field studies and measuring positive animals, using it for studying antigens, and using it for studying protection.   It seems to me, in listening to the discussion, that it is not sufficiently clear which antigens are being used.   If one does not know the protecting antigen and the protecting antibody, one worker might measure something quite different from another if he extracts the cells a little differently for getting the antigen.   If you are not working with defined antigens then I think there is no doubt that the ELISA is not very specific - it is detecting an antigen that might not agree at all with the protecting antigen, with the glycoprotein, or with the antibody which is protecting the animal.

<u>V. Moennig</u>   That is right.   Of course you are measuring different antibodies with the serum neutralisation test and the ELISA.   However, the objective in our study was just to see whether there are some Aujeszky virus specific antibodies, no matter what kind of antibodies.   In this respect I think the test is specific - specific for antibodies which are detecting some of these 20 to 30 proteins.   That is the point in our case because we have whole virus coupled to the plates and not the individual glycoproteins.

<u>H. Ludwig</u>   I think perhaps that in the long term one should try to specify the ELISA more, as the Danes do, for example, with herpes simplex diagnosis.   They really get a column-fractionated major antigen coupled to an ELISA plate and then check for the main antibody, instead of using an undefined mixture of all the antigens.

<u>K. Dalsgaard</u>   *(Denmark)*   I would like to ask why you, Dr. Toma, have chosen the ELISA system by absorbing the antigen to the plate.   To me it seems to be a relatively expensive way of using your antigen.   In human herpes virus diagnosis, people have tended to use catching antibody from another species to absorb

to the plate in the first run. There you could use either polyvalent antibodies or antibody specific to some structures mentioned by Dr. Ludwig. This is a very inexpensive way because it requires much less antigen and the antibodies can be obtained in a much easier way than large preparations of the specific types of antigen you were mentioning. I wonder why this has not been introduced into Aujeszky virus diagnosis because it is very widespread compared to many other diseases.

B. Toma   I do not think that the preparation of antigen for the ELISA in relation to AD is very expensive because when you have infected cells, centrifugation and a solution of potassium chloride, you can prepare a large amount of antigen. In our laboratory in France we have prepared sufficient antigen for 300 000 reactions in one batch.

P. Vannier (France)   On that subject, we have compared costs of the serum neutralisation test against the ELISA and in some cases we have found the ELISA to be five times less expensive.

Dr. Toma, why don't you keep your microplates at $20^{\circ}C$ below zero?

B. Toma   Simply because it is easier to have them at + $4^{\circ}C$. Also, we can sensitise plates each month, for example. We do not have to sensitise all plates for one year.

I would like to ask Dr. Moennig a question about the expression of results. When you give the titre of the serum, what is the criterion you are using?

V. Moennig   We measure the optical density at 405 nm between both wells, control well and antigen well. When the difference between these two optical densities is greater than 0.2 we consider this dilution to be positive. It is not unlike your system - you multiply that by 10 to give you your index.

B. Toma   Yes, but for your expression of results you must make the dilution?

V. Moennig   Yes, the final serum dilution which yields a difference greater than 0.2 is positive.

R.J. Lorenz   How do you arrive at the figure of 0.2?

<u>V. Moennig</u>   By comparing antigen and control wells at the wavelength of 405 nm in an apparatus comparable to Dr. Toma's.

<u>P.W. de Leeuw</u>   *(Netherlands)*   I do not want to be cynical or to discourage you but two years ago our group published on ELISA and AD. First we compared it with the one hour test and concluded that it was more sensitive than that. We then compared it with the 24 hour test and it was approximately of the same sensitivity, perhaps a little more sensitive. And yet we have stopped using the test, for various reasons. One is that within each system, as Dr. Ludwig was saying, you have to check that what you are measuring is really important in terms of protection. Secondly, we found that if we hyperimmunised animals and then took the sera, which we had checked before and afterwards, there were differences in the positive : negative ratios. The third reason was that having more confidence in the neutralisation test, we felt that it was not that difficult for a normal virological laboratory which has automated the system to a certain extent.

<u>M. Pensaert</u>   I believe that Dr. Moennig has provided the answer to Dr. de Leeuw's first point. We are not measuring protecting antibodies; it is just a matter of diagnosis. Whatever antibodies you are measuring, as long as they are formed against ADV, that is sufficient.

<u>V. Moennig</u>   It is a matter of herd diagnosis first; and secondly, as I said, I am convinced that the ELISA can be carried out by relatively unskilled persons, whereas the neutralisation test cannot be carried out by that kind of person because handling cells is much more difficult than doing the ELISA.

<u>P.W. de Leeuw</u>   I am not so sure about that. We have had quite a lot of experience with the ELISA and I am not convinced that it can be handled by inexperienced operators. Nor am I convinced that when you test a number of sera there will never be non-specific reactions. I think Dr. Gielkens might add something to that.

<u>A.L.J. Gielkens</u> *(Netherlands)*   We have checked a number of systems. When you are checking, say, 500 000 sera you will see

some non-specific reactors but it is lower than 1%. The reason
for that is not known.

Dr. Dalsgaard said that you can use a more specific
system, for example, by coupling the antibody to the well and
then catch the antigen. The problem with that system is that
you need very high titre sera. The difficulty is to get a
direct test that is as sensitive as the indirect test which is
used by Dr. Moennig and Dr. Toma. There is no problem for herd
screening but it can be a problem in an eradication programme.

B. Toma   In your system, do you compare between control antigen and viral antigen, when you test all sera?

A.L.J. Gielkens   No.

B. Toma   I think this is important because if you have both
antigens you can have with some sera a very high optical
density with control antigen but it does not matter because
you have a similar optical density with viral antigen.

H. Ludwig   Dr. Bitsch: concerning the neutralisation test,
how do you correct for the inactivation of ADV during those
24 hours? You say it is very stable, but if you work with a
small number of plaques, let's say 100 plaque forming units, I
would say that in 24 hours you reduce it to 5 or 10 plaques,
and this small number is the sensitive unit that one should
use.

V. Bitsch   We tested the thermal inactivation of our virus
clone that we used in our routine serum neutralisation test.
We compared $37^{\circ}C$ with $30^{\circ}C$ and after 18, 24 and 30 hours there
was no significant decrease in virus titre after incubation at
those two temperatures. Even after 48 hours the decrease in
virus titre was not more than 1 $\log_{10}$. That was our ordinary
virus stock. Then we thought that if we prepared our virus
stock even more carefully we could preserve the virus even
better at $37^{\circ}C$. I did not show the results because you would
not believe them! We could not detect any inactivation of the
virus at $37^{\circ}C$ for 48 hours. We harvested the virus three
hours after that maintenance medium had been changed. We did
not want to have 'old' virus particles in our stock of virus

suspension. Then again after three hours we replaced the
medium and harvested those two medium changes and used it.
Our routine stock has been thawed out and frozen down again
twice. It was certainly satisfactory.

H. Ludwig   This is a crucial point.

V. Bitsch   We used 1.5 or 2% bovine serum that we knew would
not non-specifically inactivate the virus. Perhaps that is an
important point.

H. Ludwig   There is another important point. I believe that
in the tests that you are using for diagnosis you are using
guinea pig complement. What is the situation *in vivo*? Does
the swine complement act somehow in this test; did you ever
test it *in vitro*?

V. Bitsch   Yes, we tested swine serum and calf serum and we
had a permutation of those two serum preparations. There were
differences but I don't remember which one was lower. Results
have been published on the complement-dependent neutralisation
reaction on IBR virus showing exactly the same; that complement
from other species such as the guinea pig would be sufficient.

P.W. de Leeuw   I have a comment on the 24 hour, 37°C test.
We have used it now for a couple of years in the laboratory
without any difficulty. With our strains, the Northern Ireland
strains, we have about 50% loss of virus sensitivity over the
24 hours. We aim at 200 $TCID_{50}$ and we end up with approximately
100.

The other point is that we checked it on a few hundred
sera from a minimal disease herd. It is very rare that there
are sera which react positively with a 1 in 2 or 1 in 4
dilution in these 24 hour tests. It is different in cattle.
It is now known that there are a number of cross reactions
within the herpes viruses, especially in cattle. I would not
like to recommend it just like that for cattle. We checked
about 25 SPF calves raised in complete isolation with the
24 hour test and we found that 3 of those had titres of 1 in
8 which should have been negative.

Rosalind Gaskell *(UK)* May I ask whether anyone has used class-specific ELISAs to study the development of Aujeszky immunity? Also, may I ask Dr. Terpstra whether he used coculture or explant techniques to try to detect virus in the vaccine experiment where he did not get any back from the nervous tissue?

C. Terpstra *(Netherlands)* The virus isolation was done by preparing 10% suspensions of the tissues; we did not use any explant techniques or cocultivation. I realise that these may be more sensitive than just preparing suspensions. What we tried to do was to mimic the diagnostic tests which are used in the field.

Rosalind Gaskell It is really that you got very low positive results with another of your strains of virus. You got very low titres in your tissues and therefore, presumably, it is possible that you were missing some.

C. Terpstra That was the vaccine, of course.

H. Ludwig If you are trying to prove that the vaccine strain does not go into latency by your tests, trying to assay the virus just by putting on suspension, I would very much disagree, because it is known that only by cocultivation can you get herpes virus out of a nervous system. Maybe the implications are too strong.

C. Terpstra This implication has not been made at all. I do not want to give the wrong impression. We were simply trying to check whether animals that had been vaccinated could be diagnosed by conventional methods. I agree that if you want to check whether the vaccine strains will give persistent infections, you must use quite different techniques.

B. Liess *(Federal Republic of Germany)* Before we finish this discussion session I would like to suggest that at this meeting we should try to make some proposals for standardisation of techniques, on serum neutralisation and ELISA for example. Perhaps we could form a group which could discuss such proposals.

<u>B. Toma</u>   I think it would be a good idea to form a small
working group to study this question.   Perhaps then this group
could present some conclusions and recommendations before the
end of the meeting.

(A small working group was formed)

REPORT OF THE WORKING GROUP

<u>B. Toma</u> *(France)* I would like to give you the conclusions
arrived at by the small working group which had a meeting yes-
terday afternoon.

The small working group recognised:

1) The necessity of standardisation of the results for
serological diagnosis of AD.

2) That it is impossible for all laboratories to use
exactly the same techniques with the same cell strain, the same
strain of virus, etc.

3) That different techniques with different sensitivities
will continue to be used but that it is desirable for all laboratories to have a reference serum available to compare the
sensitivity of their tests. For the definition of this reference serum, samples (including the French reference serum) will
be sent to the various laboratories represented at this meeting.
They will be tested in the same way as for a field specimen
using the seroneutralisation and any other technique routinely
used for serological diagnosis of AD. From the results of this
study a European reference serum will be proposed.

These are the conclusions and I would like to know if
everyone here agrees with these conclusions of the small working
group? If anyone here needs more information I will be glad to
answer any questions.

<u>K. Dalsgaard</u> *(Denmark)* When do you expect to send the sera?

<u>B. Toma</u> I think that the sera could be sent in about two weeks.
The sera will be diluted in normal pig sera, that is to say, in
negative pig sera - about 1 ml for each sample and about 6
samples for each laboratory. If there are participants at this
meeting who know laboratories in their own countries which would
be interested but are not represented here perhaps they could
give me their names and addresses.

<u>M. Pensaert</u> *(Belgium)* Have these sera been inactivated?

<u>B. Toma</u> I think we must decide whether it would be better to
have inactivated serum or not. What would you prefer? Has

anyone a preference? Perhaps it is better to have inactivated serum - it will be mentioned in the letter that all the sera have been inactivated.

H. Ludwig *(Federal Republic of Germany)* I think it is a good idea to have it centrally inactivated. How are you going to send it - freeze dried?

B. Toma It will be sent in liquid form. In previous studies we received good results from laboratories far from France, e.g. Czechoslovakia and Hungary, with transportation taking perhaps 4, 5 or 6 days. Even with some days at room temperature there were no problems. So I believe there is no problem in using airmail that will take a few days. In our laboratory, each time that we do this kind of study we use sera that have been kept for up to a week at room temperature.

H. Ludwig Are they absolutely sterile?

B. Toma I cannot be sure that they are all absolutely sterile. I think we should work nearer to field sera and this is certainly not completely sterile.

F. Cancellotti *(Italy)* I would like to know if we must add complement for serum neutralisation, or is this a matter of choice?

B. Toma This study is not a competition to have the highest sensitivity, to get the best results, etc. The objective is to study these sera in exactly the same way in which you always study sera, that is as a routine diagnosis. So, if you normally use complement, use it in this case, if not, do not use it. We need to know the level of sensitivity in the various laboratories in relation to their normal serological diagnosis.

B. Liess *(Federal Republic of Germany)* I was wondering why this group thinks that it is not possible or not necessary to have one common test, virus strain, or perhaps even to use similar cells?

B. Toma Within the next year or two there may well be 40 laboratories within the Community carrying out serological diagnosis of AD. Experience with other diseases has shown that it is

not possible for them all to use exactly the same technique -
with the same strain of virus, with the same strain of cell
culture, with the same doses of virus, with the same incubation
time between serum and virus, and so on. Each laboratory, or
each country, will have its own preferences. The most important
thing is to have good results - a good level of sensitivity.
If it is shown that a few laboratories do not have a good level
of sensitivity then it will be necessary to discover where the
problem lies in those cases; whether it is the virus strain,
the cell culture, the dose level or whatever. I do not think
it is realistic to expect exactly the same techniques in 40 or
50 different laboratories. In the future we may be able to move
towards standardised techniques but at the beginning of the project I think we must accept that each laboratory will use its
own technique.

Now, may I ask whether there is any disagreement in the
meeting about the conclusions of the working group, or do all
participants agree with this conclusion? Yes? Thank you.

SESSION III

PATHOGENESIS AND IMMUNITY

Chairman: A. Baskerville

CELLULAR IMMUNITY IN AUJESZKY'S DISEASE

A. Baskerville

Public Health Laboratory Service,
Centre for Applied Microbiology and Research,
Porton Down, Salisbury, Wiltshire, UK.

ABSTRACT

The roles of cell-mediated and humoral immunity in Aujeszky's disease (AD) in the pig are discussed, with particular reference to the responses following vaccination with the live avirulent Bartha strain of virus. Maximal lymphocyte stimulation was seen with cells from nodes draining the vaccination site on day 7, but this was much reduced by day 25. Responsive blood lymphocytes appeared on day 7 and were optimally stimulated on days 14 - 19. Neutralising antibody was not present on day 7 and only low titres were evident from day 14 onwards. In contrast, antibody-dependent cell-mediated cytotoxicity (ADCC) was demonstrable in some pigs on day 7 and very high titres developed by day 14 and later. It is suggested that ADCC is a very sensitive test for immunity in the pig and could be used for monitoring the immune status of herds.

Immunity to Aujeszky's disease (AD) in pigs develops after natural infection and usually confers good protection against re-infection. This immunity can be demonstrated by the presence of serum antibody, both IgG and IgM, and of IgA at mucous surfaces such as the nasal mucosa and intestine. Serum neutralising antibody to Aujeszky's disease virus (ADV) appears about 7 days after infection with virulent virus and reaches a peak after approximately 5 weeks (McFerran and Dow, 1965; McFerran and Dow, 1973). It then persists for many months (Skoda et al., 1963). The mode of infection of the pig with ADV and the pathogenesis of the disease are important in relation to vaccination methods in the control of AD. Antibody circulating in serum is active in neutralising virus which gains entry to the blood and tissue fluids. However, since the route of natural infection is usually via the nasopharynx (Baskerville et al., 1973), repulsion of the virus from these mucous membranes is probably the critical factor in preventing infection. Some IgG antibody passes across from blood vessels into the tissue fluids and even to the surface, and IgA present in nasopharyngeal secretions is also very important. The IgA peak, however, is short lived and some weeks after infection the

G. Wittmann, S.A. Hall (eds), Aujeszky's Disease. ISBN-13:978-94-009-7555-2

secretions do not contain adequate levels of anti-ADV IgA. Re-infection does stimulate the replication of clones of plasma cell precursors which mature and produce IgA.

The other defence mechanism which operates at the mucosal surface in the nose and pharynx, as well as in blood and tissues, is cell-mediated immunity (CMI). CMI is known to be important in protection against some other herpes virus infections, such as herpes simplex in man (Wilton et al., 1972; Jacob et al., 1976) and infectious bovine rhinotracheitis (IBR) in cattle (Davies and Carmichael, 1973; Rouse and Babiuk, 1974). It has been shown to function in AD in pigs by Wittman et al. (1976) and by Ashworth et al. (1979). Evidence for the existence of CMI in AD was initially circumstantial and was suggested by the fact that successful immunisation of pigs with live, avirulent strains of ADV was associated with only low levels of serum neutralising antibody (Skoda et al., 1964; McFerran and Dow, 1975). Later this was confirmed by the demonstration in pigs that the classical indicators of CMI, lymphocyte transformation and macrophage migration inhibition, were present (Wittman et al., 1976; Wittman, 1976; Ashworth et al., 1979).

The sequence of events after infection of a pig or after intranasal administration of live vaccine is as follows. Virus penetrates nasal epithelial cells and reaches the deeper tissue layers where it encounters macrophages and T-lymphocytes. Macrophages and T-lymphocytes are known to interact rapidly (macrophages producing, for example, lymphocyte-activating factor), the macrophages enhancing T-lymphocyte sensitisation and responses to antigen (Keller, 1975; Zinkernagel et al., 1980). Macrophages phagocytose some ADV antigen, and virus antigen bound to macrophage cell membrane is known to be more immunogenic than antigen alone (Pearson and Raffel, 1971). The exposure has thus primed a population of lymphocytes, and if a challenge or re-infection were to occur the lymphocytes would now be found to be capable of transformation.

The process of lymphocyte transformation (LT) produces specifically immune cells, sensitised lymphocytes, which are then able to mediate the functions of CMI *in vivo*. When

lymphocytes transform they enlarge, their synthesis of RNA
and DNA increases, and they undergo multiple divisions which
give rise to further lymphocyte populations with similar
sensitisation and properties. LT can be monitored by quantitative demonstration of incorporation of radiolabelled
precursors of DNA such as ^{3}H-thymidine. LT correlates well
with delayed hypersensitivity skin reactions. Pigs immune to
ADV have a positive skin test to ADV and their peripheral
blood T-lymphocytes transform *in vitro* when exposed to ADV
(Skoda et al., 1968; Wittmann et al., 1976; Ashworth et al.,
1979).

When they have been sensitised to ADV antigen some of
the populations of T-lymphocytes become long-lived 'memory'
cells which circulate in the blood and lymphatics and reside
in lymphnodes for several years. These cells are specifically
committed and will respond only to ADV antigen. They are
responsible for the rapid and increased CMI response on
re-exposure to ADV infection.

Following re-exposure to ADV, i.e. challenge in a
vaccinated pig, specifically sensitised T-lymphocytes function
in several ways;

1.   They produce a variety of soluble substances known as
     lymphokines; these include macrophage migration inhibition
     factor (MIF), mitogenic factor (MF), macrophage activation
     factor (MAF), leukocyte chemotactic factor (LCF), lympho-
     toxins and interferon.

2.   They directly lyse other host cells bearing ADV antigen
     on their surface - a cytolytic effect.

Lymphokines are released at the site of virus entry.
These substances greatly increase the immune response, by
inducing lymphocytes to undergo transformation and proliferation
and by recruiting more cells to the site (Rocklin et al., 1974).
In this manner the major cell types necessary for effective
resistance to AD are mobilised and activated at the sites in
which virus appears.

Cell-mediated cytolysis or cytotoxicity is the term used
to denote the capacity of some populations of sensitised
T-lymphocytes (Killer cells) to lyse directly cells which bear

those specific antigens on their surface (Lovchik and Hong, 1977). Lymphocytes in a pig immunised against ADV are sensitised to ADV and will recognise its antigen on cells and lyse them. This limits virus spread and arrests the infection. Lysis of virus-carrying cells is not only a property of specifically sensitised lymphocytes, but can also be performed by unsensitised lymphocytes, macrophages and polymorphonuclear leucocytes (PMN) if they are in the presence of antibody (Grewal et al., 1977; Russell and Miller, 1978). This provides an important link between the humoral and cellular arms of the immune response and greatly increases its effectiveness. This type of cytolysis is known as antibody-dependent cell-mediated cytotoxicity (ADCC). Since antibody is required in the system in only minute quantities it can be used as a diagnostic test for determining the level of antibody in serum and is much more sensitive than the serum neutralisation test (SNT). Unlike the enzyme-linked immunosorbent assays (ELISA), ADCC is actually demonstrating a facet of the pig's immune mechanisms and status.

The basis of the ADCC test is that various dilutions of unknown sera are mixed in microtitre plates with ADV-infected target cells, such as Vero of pig kidney, which have been radiolabelled with ^{51}Cr. Effector cells, which may be lymphocytes, macrophages or PMN are then added and they lyse virus-bearing target cells in proportion to the quantity of antibody present. This releases the ^{51}Cr from the cells and this is measured on a gamma counter. The practical details of the application of the ADCC test to AD in the pig have been described by Ashworth et al. (1979).

The recent spread of AD in pigs in Europe and its increased economic importance has led to more intensive efforts to improve vaccination and control of the disease. For this a better understanding of the protective immune response in the pig after vaccination and more sensitive methods for detection of vaccinal antibody are needed. The following summarised experimental findings were intended to contribute to this. The methods and techniques for the preparation of ADV and lymphocytes, and for measuring lymphocyte stimulation, ADCC and virus neutralisation were as described previously (Ashworth et al., 1979).

Twelve pigs were vaccinated intramuscularly (i.m.) by injection of 1 ml of Bartha ADV ($10^{6.7}$ TCD$_{50}$/ml) in the posterior aspect of the right thigh. Six control pigs were given uninfected Vero cell antigen. One week after i.m. vaccination the cells of the draining superficial and deep inguinal nodes of the Bartha pigs yielded large numbers of cells and showed a high level of stimulation. Contralateral lymphnodes yielded many fold fewer cells and showed no response. There was also no response in submandibular nodes at this stage, though splenic and blood lymphocytes gave moderate responses.

At day 14 the draining inguinal nodes provided only about twice as many cells as the contralaterals and the response was slightly reduced. Blood lymphocytes in all pigs gave higher levels of stimulation than at 7 days, but submandibular node and spleen cells were the same as day 7.

Between days 25 and 27 after vaccination, the draining inguinal and contralateral nodes were of similar size and gave similarly modest stimulation responses. Submandibular node cells gave similar results, though blood lymphocyte responses had increased still further.

By SNT, no antibody was detectable on day 7 in any vaccinated pig (Table 1) and only low titres were apparent at 14 and 25 - 27 days. Control sera had no virus neutralising activity.

In vaccinated pigs anti-viral ADCC was detected at low titre in 2 pigs on day 7 (Table 1). By day 14 ADCC titres were high in all 4 test pigs and were even higher on days 25 - 27. The much greater sensitivity of the ADCC test as compared with SNT can be seen from the figures in Table 1.

These results show that one week after i.m. immunisation of pigs with a live vaccine strain of ADV the draining inguinal lymphnodes contain cells capable of considerable *in vitro* secondary responses to ADV antigen. Coupled with the observed increase in cellularity of the nodes this implies the generation of great potential for response to subsequent challenge *in vivo*. At 7 days also blood and spleen cells showed some degree of lymphocyte sensitivity. A decline in

TABLE 1

ANTIBODY RESPONSES OF PIGS VACCINATED WITH THE BARTHA STRAIN OF ADV

Pig	Days after vaccination	Serum antibody titre neutralising	ADCC
A)		−	−
B)	7	−	32
G)		−	16
H)		−	−
D)		8	1 024
E)	14	4	2 048
K)		4	1 024
L)		8	2 048
N)	25	4	4 096
O)		8	1 024
Q)	27	16	4 096
R)		8	2 048

sensitivity of cells from the draining nodes was complemented
by the appearance of detectable responses in submandibular and
contralateral inguinal node lymphocytes, and an increase in
blood lymphocyte reactivity. These findings differ slightly
from those of Wittmann (1976) using virulent infection of
pigs, in that this author had found no significant blood
lymphocyte responses at any time. Lymphocyte stimulation,
however, has been demonstrated frequently using blood cells in
herpes virus diseases of other species (Rouse and Babiuk, 1974;
Rosenberg and Notkins, 1974; Thomson and Mumford, 1977).

A comparison of serum neutralisation and ADCC titres
showed values consistently many times higher for ADCC, and very
low SN levels, which in the field would have been difficult
to interpret. Similar results have also been obtained using
the guinea pig as a model for AD in other species (Ashworth
et al., 1980). The ADCC test is no more cumbersome to perform
than SNT if a laboratory is equipped for radiolabelling and
counting. We feel that ADCC could be extremely useful as a
herd serological test for AD in pigs, because of its very high
sensitivity and its ability to detect as positive pigs which
are negative to the SNT or have low and doubtful SN titres.
Further investigation of the method is worthwhile, since it may

have application in detecting latent infection in carrier pigs.
The ADCC test provides information about mechanisms of the
immune response to ADV and is thus also valuable as a research
tool.

REFERENCES

Ashworth, L.A.E., Lloyd, G. and Baskerville, A., 1979. Antibody-dependent
    cell-mediated cytotoxicity (ADCC) in Aujeszky's disease. Arch.
    Virol., 59, 307-318.
Ashworth, L.A.E., Baskerville, A. and Lloyd, G., 1980. Aujeszky's disease
    in the guinea pig: cellular and humoral responses following immun-
    ization. Arch. Virol., 63, 227-237.
Baskerville, A., McFerran, J.B. and Dow, C., 1973. Aujeszky's disease in
    pigs. Vet. Bull., 43, 465-480.
Davies, D.H. and Carmichael, L.E., 1973. Role of cell-mediated immunity in
    the recovery of cattle from primary and recurrent infections with
    infectious bovine rhinotracheitis virus. Infect. Immun., 8, 510-518.
Grewal, A.S., Rouse, B.T. and Babiuk, L.A., 1977. Mechanisms of resistance
    to herpesviruses: comparison of the effectiveness of different cell
    types in mediating antibody-dependent cell-mediated cytotoxicity.
    Infect. Immun., 15, 698-707.
Jacobs, R.P., Aurelian, L. and Cole, G.A., 1976. Cell-mediated immune
    response to Herpes simplex virus. J. Immunol., 116, 1520-1525.
Keller, R., 1975. Major changes in lymphocyte proliferation evoked by
    activated macrophages. Cell Immunol., 17, 542-547.
Lovchik, J.C. and Hong, R., 1977. Antibody-dependent cell-mediated cyto-
    lysis (ADCC): analysis and projections. Progr. Allergy. 22, 1-44.
McFerran, J.B. and Dow, C., 1965. The distribution of the virus of
    Aujeszky's disease (pseudorabies virus) in experimentally infected
    swine. Amer. J. vet. Res., 26, 631-636.
McFerran, J.B. and Dow, C., 1973. The effect of colostrum-derived
    antibody on mortality and virus excretion following experimental
    infection of piglets with Aujeszky's disease virus. Res. vet. Sci.,
    15, 208-214.
McFerran, J.B. and Dow, C., 1975. Studies on immunization of pigs with
    the Bartha strain of Aujeszky's disease virus. Res. vet. Sci., 19,
    17-22.
Pearson, M.N. and Raffel, S., 1971. Macrophage-digested antigen as inducer
    of delayed hypersensitivity. J. exp. Med., 133, 494-501.
Rocklin, R.E., MacDermott, R.P., Chess, L., Schlossman, S.F. and David,
    J.R., 1974. Studies on mediator production by highly purified
    human T and B lymphocytes. J. exp. Med., 140, 1303-1316.
Rosenberg, G.L. and Notkins, A.L., 1974. Induction of cellular immunity
    to herpes simplex virus: relationship to the humoral immune response.
    J. Immunol., 112, 1019-1025.
Rouse, B.T. and Babiuk, L.A., 1974. Host defence mechanisms against
    infectious bovine rhinotracheitis virus: in vitro stimulation of
    sensitized lymphocytes by virus antigen. Infect. Immun., 10, 681-686.
Russell, A.S. and Miller, C., 1978. A possible role for polymorpho-
    nuclear leucocytes in the defence against recrudescent herpes simplex
    virus infection in man. Immunology, 34, 371-378.
Skoda, R., Sadecky, E. and Molnar, J., 1963. Über die bei Mutterschweinen
    nach natürlicher Infektion serologisch nachweisbare Immunität gegen
    die Aujeszkysche Krankheit. Arch. exp. Vet. Med., 17, 1363-1370.

Skoda, R., Brauner, I., Sadecky, E. and Somogyiova, J., 1964. Immunization against Aujeszky's disease with live vaccine. II. Immunization of pigs under laboratory conditions. Acta. virol., 8, 123-134.

Skoda, R., Ivanicova, S., Jamrichova, O. and Sliepka, M., 1968. Die kutane Überempfindlichkeit der Schweine bei Aujeszkyscher Krankheit. Arch. exp. Vet. Med., 22, 925-936.

Thomson, G.R. and Mumford, J.A., 1977. *In vitro* stimulation of foal lymphocytes with equid herpes virus. Res. vet. Sci. 22, 347-352.

Wilton, J.M.A., Ivanyi, L. and Lehner, T., 1972. Cell-mediated immunity in Herpesvirus hominis infections. Br. Med. J., 1, 723-726.

Wittmann, G., 1976. Cell-mediated immunity in Aujeszky disease virus infected pigs. II. Influence of lymphocytes on macrophage migration Zbl. Vet. Med. B 23, 520-528.

Wittmann, G., Bartenbach, G. and Jakubik, J., 1976. Cell-mediated immunity in Aujeszky disease virus infected pigs. I. Lymphocytic stimulation. Arch. Virol., 50, 215-222.

Zinkergagel, R.M., Kreeb, G. and Althage, A., 1980. Lymphohemopoietic origin of the immunogenic virus-antigen-presenting cells triggering anti-viral T-cell responses. Clin. Immunol. Immunopath., 15, 565-576.

PRECIPITATING ANTIGENS INVOLVED IN PROTECTION AGAINST AUJESZKY'S DISEASE AFTER NATURAL INFECTION AND AFTER IMMUNISATION WITH INACTIVATED VACCINE

K. Dalsgaard.

State Veterinary Institute for Virus Research
Lindholm, DK-4771 Kalvehave, Denmark.

ABSTRACT

It was shown by crossed immunoelectrophoresis that Aujeszky virus produced a similar precipitating antigen profile as previously described for herpes hominis virus.

Intranasal infection of pigs with the virus elicited a precipitating antibody response against several virus-specific antigens, whereas vaccination of pigs with an inactivated Aujeszky vaccine produced a more restricted precipitin response, mainly directed against viral glycoproteins.

Guinea pigs immunised with preparations containing glycoproteins derived from Triton X 100 treated infected cells developed neutralising antibodies and were resistant to challenge.

A detergent treated Aujeszky antigen preparation was used successfully for the detection of serum antibodies by immunoelectro-osmophoresis.

INTRODUCTION

Characterisation of herpes hominis virus antigens by crossed immunoelectrophoresis was originally reported by Faber Vestergaard (1973). Using the same system we are describing here the antigen profile of the Aujeszky virus.

The effect of vaccination against Aujeszky's disease with an inactivated vaccine has been compared to the effect of natural infection by Jakubik et al. (1978). Using sera from these animals we are reporting here on the difference in precipitating antibodies between the two groups, using crossed immunoelectrophoresis. Furthermore, we are describing the protective effect of a detergent split Aujeszky antigen product in a guinea pig challenge model.

Finally, the use of this antigen for the serological diagnosis of Aujeszky's disease in pigs by immunoelectro-osmophoresis is reported.

G. Wittmann, S.A. Hall (eds), Aujeszky's Disease. ISBN-13:978-94-009-7555-2

MATERIALS AND METHODS

Crossed immunoelectrophoresis

The method of Weeke (1973) was used. Details including the use of Concanavalin A intermediate gel have been described in previous publications (Bøg-Hansen, 1973; Dalsgaard, 1977).

Aujeszky antigen

Primary pig kidney monolayer cell cultures were infected with a Danish isolate of Aujeszky virus at a multiplicity of infection of 10 : 1. After 24 h the cells were scraped off the glass wall and precipitated by centrifugation. The cell pellet was suspended in 3 volumes of 10% Triton x 100 in 0.01 M Tris buffer pH 7.5. After sonication the mixture was ultracentrif-uged at 100 000 x g for 1 h. The supernatant was used as antigen throughout, and is referred to as Aujeszky antigen (AA).

Sera

For characterisation of the antigen profile a hyperimmune pig serum obtained by repeated intranasal inoculations with Aujeszky virus was used (Bitsch and Eskildsen, 1976).

Ten pig sera taken 2 weeks after natural infection, and 10 pig sera taken 2 weeks after revaccination with an inactivated vaccine (Jakubik and Wittmann, 1978) were kindly provided by Professor Wittmann, Tübingen.

Guinea pig sera were obtained after subcutaneous inoculation of 10 guinea pigs with AA, 3 x 50 μl in an equal volume of Freund's incomplete adjuvant at 2 week intervals. The sera were screened for precipitating antibodies against AA by crossed immunoelectrophoresis. Sera showing strong reaction against a major antigen were pooled and re-electrophoresed against AA.

Precipitin lines of the major antigen were cut from the plates and emulsified in Freund's incomplete adjuvant (1 line/ 0.1 ml). Ten guinea pigs were immunised with 0.3 ml of this preparation 3 times at 2 week intervals. Ten days after the last inoculation sera were collected and the animals were subjected to challenge with 100 GPLD$_{50}$ units of Aujeszky virus, as were 10 controls.

Vaccination experiment

Serial 4-fold dilutions of AA were used to immunise 5 groups of 8 guinea pigs. A dose of undiluted vaccine given to the first group consisted of AA corresponding to a nitrogen content of 100 µg estimated according to Lowry et al. (1951) in a dose volume of 0.5 ml made up in PBS. Serial dilutions were made in PBS.

A duplicate group of 5 x 8 guinea pigs received the same dilutions of AA, with the addition of 50 µg of the adjuvant Quil A (Dalsgaard, 1978) for each animal. These animals and ten controls were challenged four weeks after vaccination with 100 GPLD$_{50}$ units of Aujeszky virus. As soon as clinical symptoms appeared the diseased animals were killed.

Immunoelectro-osmophoresis

Details will be published elsewhere.

RESULTS

Figure 1 shows the crossed electrophoresis of Triton x 100 solubilised Aujeszky virus infected cells (AA) against hyperimmune pig serum (15 µl against 0.5 ml). At least 8 distinct arcs can be seen. Control runs with mock infected cells against the same serum or AA antigen against normal pig serum did not show any precipitation.

Ten sera received from Professor G. Wittman, Tübingen, from experimentally infected pigs produced essentially the same pattern e.g. from 6 to 9 arcs could be detected. Ten sera also received from Professor Wittmann but taken from pigs revaccinated with an inactivated Aujeszky vaccine produced a distinctly different result. In all sera the most heavily stained arc (indicated in Figure 1 by an arrow) was detected almost exclusively. Only a few minor arcs in two of the sera could be seen. An example of crossed electrophoreses of the post-vaccination sera is given in Figure 2 left.

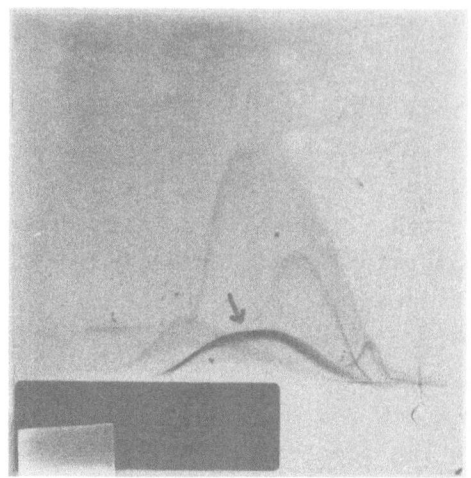

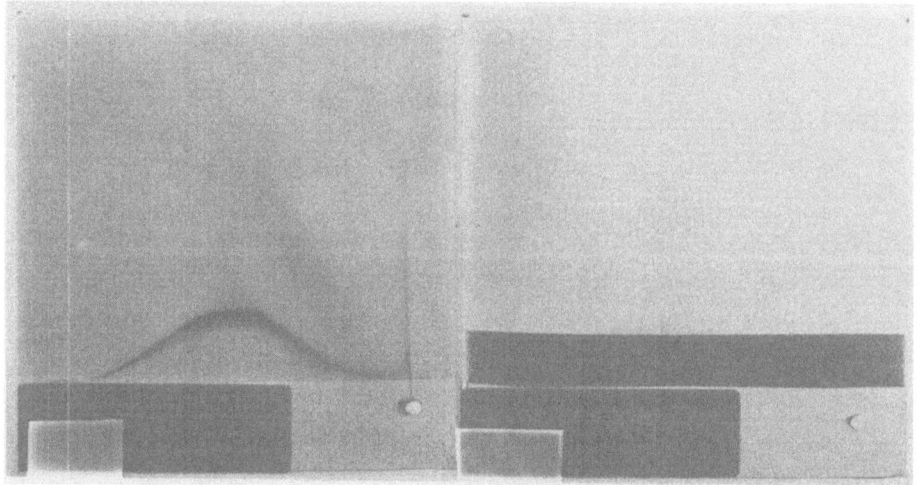

Fig. 2.

By introduction of an intermediate gel containing Concanavalin A it was demonstrated that the antigen(s) in this
major arc had binding affinity to the lectin, indicating that
the antigen(s) were of glycoprotein nature (Figure 2 right).

By immunising guinea pigs with AA, precipitating antibodies to this major glycoprotein antigen(s) were produced
after only two injections, but antibodies to a few other antigens were also seen. The major precipitin arc was excised for
the repeated inoculation of 10 other guinea pigs and these

animals produced serum antobodies only reacting with the glycoprotein antigen(s), (Figure 3).

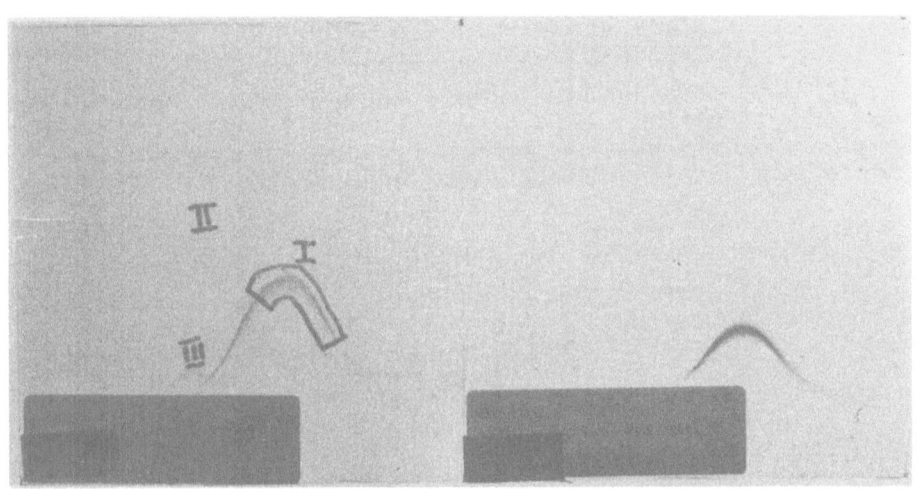

These sera all showed neutralising capacity against
Aujeszky virus higher than 1 : 32 as tested in monolayer cell
culture tubes (1 h - 37°C - 100 $TCID_{50}$). Furthermore, all the
animals were resistant to challenge with Aujeszky virus, whereas
10 control animals showed generalised disease after the same
challenge.

To investigate the protective capacity of a single
inoculation of AA in guinea pigs an experiment was set up using
vaccination with 4-fold dilutions of antigen. Another group
of guinea pigs was vaccinated with the same antigen dilutions,
but additionally each animal received 50 µg of the water
soluble saponin adjuvant Quil A to see if a possible protective
effect could be enhanced. The results can be seen in Figure 4.

Using a 50% protection end point for comparison, the group
without adjuvant was calculated to be protected at dilution
1 : 7. The group receiving Quil A was protected at dilution
1 : 45 indicating that the adjuvant enhanced the potency of
the vaccine about 6-fold. In addition it can be seen that
undiluted vaccine and dilution 1 : 4 induced 100% protection of
the guinea pigs when the vaccine contained Quil A. All 10
control animals showed generalised disease after challenge.

112

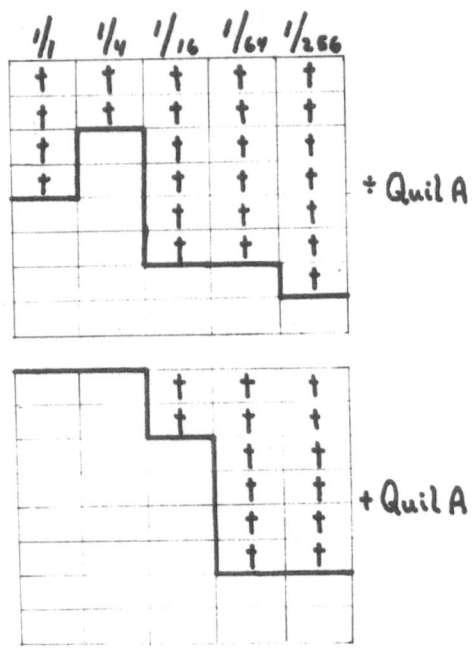

Fig. 4.

AA was tested for possible use in the serological diagnosis of Aujeszky positive sera. Since it reacted well in the
electrophoretic precipitation system, immunoelectro-osmophoresis,
or counter current electrophoresis, was tested. The results can
be seen in Figure 5.

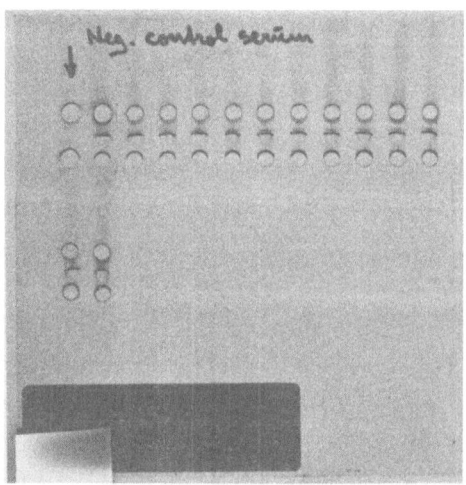

Undiluted serum samples positive for Aujeszky antibodies
in neutralisation tests were run against AA diluted 1 : 10.
Up to now relatively few sera have been tested and compared to
the results of other diagnostic techniques. However, two
experimentally infected pigs were thoroughly investigated.
Sera were taken daily and the development of antibodies was
followed by neutralisation, complement fixation (Bitsch and
Eskildsen, 1976), and immunoelectro-osmophoresis. From these
results it appeared that the latter technique detected antibodies at least as early as conventional neutralisation and
complement fixation.

DISCUSSION

Crossed immunoelectrophoresis of detergent solubilised
Aujeszky virus infected cells produced almost the same pattern
and number of detectable antigens as reported for herpes hominis virus (Faber Vestergaard, 1973). This was true when using
pig antisera obtained after natural infection. Obviously the
replication of the virus in the host elicits an immune response
to a variety of antigens. Sera taken from animals vaccinated
with an inactivated vaccine, however, showed a much more restricted antibody profile, and it was shown that these antibodies were
directed mainly against glycoprotein antigens probably located
on the surface of Aujeszky virus. It has been demonstrated by
Norrild et al. (1977) that the glycoprotein precipitation arc
in crossed immunoelectrophoresis of herpes hominis virus in a
similar system contains a complex of several antigens. This
may also be the case in our experiments with Aujeszky virus, but
it remains to be investigated by radioprecipitation techniques.

Injection of Aujeszky virus glycoprotein-(complex)
precipitation lines in guinea pigs induced neutralising antibodies and protection against challenge in the animals. These
results indicate that the presence of the glycoprotein complex
in inactivated vaccines plays a significant role for their
efficacy, and suggest that quantitative immunoelectrophoretic
techniques might be useful for the evaluation of vaccine antigens. It is not known whether the relatively restricted immune
response to inactivated vaccines is of any practical importance

but one might fear this, remembering the discouraging results
with inactivated vaccines against paramyxoviruses in humans
(Merz et al., 1980; Norrby et al., 1975); especially after the
results of Bitsch (1980) demonstrating the possibility that some
of the more virulent Aujeszky virus strains produce syncytia
in cell culture. If this is significant *in vivo*, it seems
important also to induce antibodies against this (fusion
protein?) antigen.

It was demonstrated that detergent-split Aujeszky virus
infected cells were able to induce resistance to challenge
with virus in guinea pigs, and that this effect could be
enhanced by Quil A. From a practical point of view this seems
to be an attractive new approach to the formulation of Aujeszky
vaccines. However, from our point of view the application of
vaccines in the eradication of the disease is not desirable.
Much more important is the availability of sensitive diagnostic
techniques. The immunoelectro-osmophoresis described in this
paper may represent a valuable supplementary tool. This
approach has been reported previously by Papp-Vid et al. (1978)
using aqueous virus suspensions as the antigen. In the system
described here using AA, we think that the antigen preparation
is easier and possibly exposes new antigenic sites by the
action of the detergent.

REFERENCES

Bitsch, V., 1980. Correlation between the pathogenicity of field strains
    of Aujeszky's disease virus and their ability to cause cell fusion -
    syncytia formation - in cell cultures. Acta vet. scand. 21, 708-710.
Bitsch, V. and Eskildsen, M., 1976. A comparative examination of swine
    sera for antibody to Aujeszky virus with the conventional and a
    modified virus-serum neutralisation test and a modified direct com-
    plement fixation test. Acta vet. scand. 17, 142-152.
Bøg-Hansen, T.C., 1973. Crossed immuno-affinoelectrophoresis. An
    analytical method to predict the result of affinity chromatography.
    Analyt. Biochem. 56, 480-488.
Dalsgaard, K., 1977. Crossed immunoelectrophoretic characterization of
    virus-specified antigens in cells infected with african swine fever
    virus. J. gen. Virol. 36, 203-206.
Dalsgaard, K., 1978. A study of the isolation and characterization of the
    saponin Quil A. Acta vet. scand., suppl. 69, 1-40.
Faber Vestergaard, B., 1973. Crossed immunoelectrophoretic characterization
    of herpesvirus hominis type 1 and 2 antigens. Acta path. microb.
    scand. B, 81, 808-810.

115

Jakubik, J. and Wittmann, G., 1978. Neutralizing antibody titres in pig serum after revaccination with an inactivated Aujeszky disease virus (ADV) vaccine. Zbl. vet. med. 325, 741-751.

Lowry, O.H., Rosebrough, N.I., Farr, A.L. and Randall, R.J., 1951. Protein measurement with the folin phenol reagent. J. Biol. Chem. 193, 265-275.

Merz, D.C., Scheir, A. and Choppin, P.W., 1980. Importance of antibodies to the fusion glycoprotein of paramyxoviruses in the prevention of spread of infection. J. exp. med. 151, 275-288.

Norrby, E. Enders-Ruckle, G. and ter Meulen, V., 1975. Differences in the appearance of antibodies to structural components of measles virus after immunization with inactivated and live virus. J. infect. dis. 132, 262-272.

Norrild, B. and Faber Vestergaard, B., 1977. Polyacrylamide gel electrophoretic analysis of herpes simplex virus type 1 immunoprecipitates obtained by quantitative immunoelectrophoresis in antibody containing agarose gel. J. Virol. 22, 113-117.

Papp-Vid, G. and Dulac, G.C., 1978. Pseudorabies: Adaption of the countercurrent immunoelectrophoresis for the detection of antibodies in porcine serum. Can. J. comp. med. 43, 119-124.

Weeke, B., 1973. In a manual of quantitative immunoelectrophoresis. Scand. J. Immunol. Suppl. no. 1.

EXPERIMENTAL NASAL INFECTION OF CATTLE WITH AUJESZKY'S DISEASE VIRUS (ADV)

G. Wittmann, U. Höhn, F. Weiland and H.O. Böhm

Federal Research Institute for Animal Virus Diseases,
D-7400 Tübingen, Federal Republic of Germany.

ABSTRACT

Seven calves and cows were experimentally infected with Aujeszky's disease virus (ADV) by the nasal route. The lowest virus dose used was 10^4 TCD_{50}. The clinical signs as well as the most prominent post mortem and histological findings are described. Virus distribution throughout the body was dependent on the time of death. In one calf that died on day post infection (d.p.i.) 3, virus was detected only in the nasal mucosa and in the thymus. With another calf that died on d.p.i. 5, virus was isolated from the retropharyngeal lymphnodes and the brain. With those animals that died on d.p.i. 6 or 7, virus was isolated only from the central nervous system. During the infection period from d.p.i. 1 onward ADV could regularly be isolated from the nasal secretion of the cows but not of the calves. The results are discussed with regard to the pathogenesis of ADV infection in cattle, the role of cattle as a source of infection and the inter-relation between infected pigs and cattle.

INTRODUCTION

Following the results of an experiment by McFerran and Dow in 1964, who could not detect Aujeszky's disease virus (ADV) in the nasal secretion of i.n. infected calves, it has been generally accepted that cattle are epidemiologically of no importance and cannot act as a source of infection. From the field sporadic cases have been reported where cattle have contracted Aujeszky's disease (AD) without being in the same stable as infected pigs. In one case the cattle stable was about 100 m distant from the pig house. Therefore, we decided to investigate a) the dose of ADV necessary for infection of cattle and b) the possibility of virus being shed with the nasal secretion of the infected cattle.

MATERIALS AND METHODS

Three calves that were 3, 4 and 5 weeks old, and 4 cows, 1½ years old, were infected with different doses of ADV by the nasal route. The virus dose ranged from 10^{10} to 10^4 TCD_{50}. The virus was the virulent pig strain Phylaxia, 5th passage in

BHK cell cultures. The temperature of the animals was taken daily and their clinical state observed.

During the infection period blood samples and nasal swabs were taken. After death samples were taken for virological examination from the following organs and tissues: nasal mucosa tonsils, salivary glands, retropharyngeal, cervical and inguinal lymphnodes, lung, liver, spleen, kidney, heart, transudate of the pericardial sac, vaginal mucosa, ganglion trigeminale (only with cows), olfactorial bulb, brain stem, medulla and the cervical, thoracical and lumbal part of the spinal cord. In the case of the calves the thymus was also examined. In two animals with pruritis, the affected skin region, including sub-cutis and muscles, was examined.

Virus isolations from nasal swabs and ground tissue suspensions were done in BHK cell culture tubes in tenfold dilution steps.

The sera of the animals were examined at different times after infection by the neutralisation test. This test was also used to identify the ADV isolates from the nasal swabs. The test was performed in the presence of 10% guinea pig complement according to the method previously described (Wittmann et al., 1976; Jakubik and Wittmann, 1979).

Histological studies were made with various organs of the dead animals after fixation in formalin (10%) and haemalaun-eosin staining.

RESULTS

A nasal discharge appeared in all the animals on the third day post infection (d.p.i.). Severe clinical symptoms set in either at the same time or between one and 3 days later. The incubation period was apparently dependent on the virus dose used, since it was the shortest with those animals that received 10^9 and 10^{10} TCD_{50}. However, since these animals were the youngest ones, namely 3 and 4 weeks old, the possibility that age was also an influence cannot be excluded. However, the onset of severe symptoms occurred on d.p.i. 6 in a 5 week old calf, which was inoculated with 10^8 TCD_{50}, so, the influence of age is somewhat questionable. The predominant severe symptoms

were disorder of the central nervous system, dyspnoea and
swelling of the rumen. Itching could only be observed in 2 of
the 7 animals in the head region. All the animals died within
24 hours after the onset of the nervous symptoms in a very
dramatic way. Some hours before death, the older animals, but
not the calves, had a brief fever. Severe signs of illness
were the rule; however, one calf showed only a brief and slight
reduction of appetite but nevertheless died within 12 hours
afterwards.

The most frequent *post mortem* findings were inflammation
of the nasal mucosa, alveolar oedema in the lung, hyperaemia in
the lung and brain, subendocardial, subepicardial and myocardial
haemorrhages, light spots in the heart muscle, transudate in
the pericardial sac, dry intestinal mucosa with some
haemorrhages.

Histologically we found: infiltrations of lymphocytes and
neutrophils in the myocardium, oedema and hyperaemia in the
lung, oedema in the lymphnodes, inflammatory cell infiltrates
in the mucosa of the colon. In the central nervous system there
were menigeal and perivascular infiltrations consisting of
lymphocytes and a few neutrophils; glia foci and, sometimes,
necrosis of ganglia cells.

Table 1 shows that the distribution of the virus throughout the body varied depending on the time of death. In calf no.
1 which died d.p.i. 3 virus was found only in the nasal mucosa
and the thymus. In calf no. 2 which died d.p.i. 5 virus was
detected on the retropharyngeal lymphnodes and in different
parts of the brain. With those animals which died on d.p.i. 6
or 7 (nos. 3 to 7) virus could only be isolated from different
parts of the brain and from the cervical part of the spinal
cord. Neutralising antibodies could not be detected in any of
the animals.

This virus distribution gives rise to some speculation
with regard to the pathogenesis of ADV infection in cattle.
Apparently, primary virus multiplication occurs in the
pharyngeal and nasal region during the first 3 days after i.n.
infection. The thymus may also be involved. It is striking that
no virus could be isolated from the tonsils. Primary virus

TABLE 1

ADV IN THE ORGANS OF INTRANASALLY INFECTED CATTLE

Cattle no.	Age	Dose of infect. TCD_{50}	Death d.p.i.	ND_{50}	Isolation of virus from the organs ($\log_{10}$ TCD_{50}/0.1g)							
					Nasal mucosa	Phary. Ln.	Thymus	Gangl. trigem.	Olfact. bulbus	Brain stem	Medulla	Cervical cord
1	3 weeks	10^{10}	3	-	4.1	-	3.3	n.d.	-	-	-	-
2	4	10^9	5	-	-	0.9	-	n.d.	1.9	3.3	4.5	-
3	5	10^8	7	-	-	-	-	n.d.	3.5	3.7	3.5	1.3
4	1.5 years	10^7	6	-	-	-	n.d.	2.7	2.7	5.3	4.7	2.9
5	1.5	10^6	7	-	-	-	n.d.	1.3	2.9	3.9	3.3	-
6	1.5	10^5	6	-	-	-	n.d.	1.1	1.9	3.3	3.7	0.9
7	1.5	10^4	6	-	-	-	n.d.	2.1	1.9	2.9	2.7	-

No virus isolation from tonsils, salivary glands, inguinal and cervical lymphnodes, lung, liver, spleen, heart, pericard transudate, kidney, vaginal mucosa, thoracic and lumbal cord, skin and muscles of itching area.

multiplication in cattle is apparently more limited and of shorter duration than in pigs (Wittmann et al., 1980). From the sites of primary virus multiplication the virus reaches via the nervous pathway, the olfactory bulb, the ganglion trigeminale, the brain stem, the medulla and the cervical cord. The complete failure to isolate virus from other parts of the body may indicate that in contrast to pigs (Wittmann et al., 1980), no virus distribution takes place on the haematogenic and lymphatic pathway.

Table 2 shows that ADV could regularly be isolated from the nasal secretions of the older cattle from the time of infection onward until death. This was not the case with the calves and this corresponds to the finding of McFerran and Dow (1964). A comparison of the titres after 4 hours post infection with the later ones reveals that a real virus multiplication had taken place in the nasal region. The virus excretion from cattle was significantly lower than with pigs, where we found maximum titres up to $10^{6.1}$ TCD_{50} (unpublished results). Gutekunst and Pirtle (1979) report titres up to $10^{8.3}$ TCD_{50}. Nevertheless, the level of up to $10^{3.9}$ TCD_{50} of ADV excreted by cattle and the long period of virus excretion may be sufficient for infecting other cattle or pigs.

TABLE 2

ADV IN THE NASAL SECRETION OF I.N. INFECTED CATTLE

Cattle no.	Age	Dose of infect. TCD_{50}	$\log_{10}$ TCD_{50} ADV per nasal swab, d.p.i.							
			4 h	1	2	3	4	5	6	7
1	3 weeks	10^{10}	n.d.	–	–	1.7*				
2	4	10^{9}	n.d.	–	–	–	–	*		
3	5	10^{8}	n.d.	–	–	–	–	–	–	*
4	1.5 years	10^{7}	1.7	3.3	2.7	1.9	1.9	C	*	
5	1.5	10^{6}	1.3	2.3	2.9	3.5	2.1	1.3	C	C*
6	1.5	10^{5}	1.3	3.5	3.5	2.9	3.3	1.9	1.0*	
7	1.5	10^{4}	1.5	3.1	3.9	2.3	3.3	2.9	1.1	

C = Contaminated

Therefore, the assumption that cattle can only be infected by pigs and that infected cattle are not a source of infection should be revised. The pig/cattle interaction only applies in relation to the fact that AD is usually introduced in mixed pig/cattle herds by infected pigs. Since a rather low level of ADV is sufficient to infect cattle, the possibility that ADV can be transmitted to separate cattle herds under unfavourable conditions can no longer be excluded; transmission of infection may occur through air currents over a short distance, caused by ventilators in the pig stable, by virus contaminated food and by contaminated personnel.

REFERENCES

Gutekunst, D.E. and Pirtle, E.C., 1979. Humoral and cellular immune responses in swine after vaccination with inactivated pseudorabies virus. Am. J. Vet. Res. 40, 1343-1346.
Jakubik, J. and Wittmann, G., 1979. Neutralizing antibody titres in pig serum after revaccination with an inactivated Aujeszky's disease virus (ADV) vaccine. Zbl. Vet. Med. B 325, 741-759.
McFerran, J.B. and Dow, C., 1964. Virus studies on experimental Aujeszky's disease in calves. J. Comp. Path. 74, 173-179.
Wittmann, G., Bartenbach, G. and Jakubik, J., 1976. Cell-mediated immunity in Aujeszky's disease virus infected pigs. Arch. Virol. 50, 215-222.
Wittmann, G., Jakubik, J. and Ahl, R., 1980. Multiplication and distribution of Aujeszky's disease (pseudorabies) virus in vaccinated and non-vaccinated pigs after intranasal infection. Arch. Virol. 66, 227-240.

GENERAL DISCUSSION

J.B. McFerran (UK) Professor Wittmann, could you give us
details of the virus used for inoculation. I am asking this
because I think there is a big problem arising with changes in
behaviour of Aujeszky's virus. For example, for many years we
routinely looked at faeces as well as the central nervous
system for Aujeszky's virus in pigs. It is only in the last
two years that we have occasionally found ADV in the
faeces. Was this a laboratory strain, or was it a recent
isolate? What is the passage history?

G. Wittmann (Federal Republic of Germany) The strain we used was
a virulent strain from Hungary, named Phylaxia which we got
about five years ago. It was isolated from pigs. We passaged
this virus three to four times in BHK cell cultures and then
we inoculated the cattle.

J. Th. van Oirschot (Netherlands) Dr. Baskerville, what kind
of neutralisation test did you use? How did you read the end
point of the ADCC? Thirdly, in the introduction to your talk
you gave some results on IgA in nasal washings; can you be more
precise about those results?

A. Baskerville (UK) Taking the third question first, no, this
was a general review when I was talking about IgA. We have not
studied it in any great detail; we have not followed all the
animals with nasal washings.

The serum neutralisation was just a standard 100 $TCID_{50}$
with no complement added. Incidentally, there is a totally
different system, which is complement-dependent ADCC which we
find is not as sensitive as ADCC. Complement did not enhance
the ADCC system. I can give you the details of the tests later
if you wish.

J. Th. van Oirschot Yes, thank you. Of course it is very
important which technique you use and also which end point you
use in the ADCC because there can be large variations, for
instance, in spontaneous release.

A. Baskerville   That is right. You do need a lot of controls
and we take as positive 20% over control - in other words you
have got to have greater than 20%. A lot of the work on IBR
and herpes simplex has taken 10 or 15%, and in some cases 5%.
We feel you have got to have at least 20% over and above
control systems.

J. Th. van Oirschot   Again, you can have different controls,
negative serum or negative cells.

A. Baskerville   That's right; you have to have hyperimmune
serum as a standard; you also have to have 100% release from
2% Triton-X 100 as a control. You need a lot of controls.

H. Ludwig (Federal Republic of Germany)   What cells did you use
to perform the ADCC, lymphocytes?

A. Baskerville   We have used macrophages of various origins,
and lymphocytes, and polymorphs as well. However, for a
diagnostic test you can use whole blood leukocytes for six
hours. There would be no advantage in using separated lymphocytes, macrophages or polymorphs. We were simply looking at
that to study the role of the different cell types in the
immune response. But, from a test point of view, you could
use Dextran-sedimented whole blood leukocytes, which would be
much simpler of course.

H. Ludwig   Since ADCC is known to be a very sensitive test,
how can you be sure you are not detecting some anti-mycoplasma
antibodies? What was the source of your virus and your cells?

A. Baskerville   We have never had any evidence that we had
problems with mycoplasmas. You can run into trouble if you
don't use different cell lines for vaccinating your animals,
and for the *in vitro* system. If you use the same cell line
then you will find that there is quite a high basal release,
because the animals have an immune response to the cell antigens, whether it is pig kidney or another cell line. Because

it is a very sensitive technique you are picking up antibody
to the cell fragments, cell antigens. One does have to be aware
of that.

M. Pensaert *(Belgium)*   Professor Wittmann, you have shown that
the virus is excreted in nasal secretions in cattle and you
conclude that it may be that transmission occurs to other
cattle. But did you prove that under natural circumstances,
with natural exposure?

G. Wittmann   No, we did not prove that.

M. Pensaert   It may be that the virus quantity was not high
enough, or that you need more virus in order to get the
infection started by natural exposure.

G. Wittmann   But there was excretion for between 3 and 7 days.
If you consider a virus content of 10^4 for 6 or 7 days, being
excreted all the time, I think that must be sufficient virus
in the stable to infect other animals.

M. Pensaert   Well, it all depends what the minimal quantity is
in order to get the infection started in cattle. Did you
determine that?

G. Wittmann   Yes, we used 10^4 TCD_{50}, and we succeeded, but in
a second experiment, with the same level, we did not succeed.
It is possible that this is the lower level of infection, and
that for regular infection of cattle it is necessary to use
10^5 or 10^6 TCD_{50}.

M. Pensaert   That is what I mean. In the case of natural
infection, even if you find a given amount of virus in the
nasal secretions, it might be that the animal next to the
infected one never gets that much virus to be infected with.
So, I was wondering whether your conclusion is perhaps a little
bit too strict, or a little bit too dangerous.

G. Wittmann   Each of these animals was isolated in different
stables.

V. Bitsch   *(Denmark)*   You mentioned a case of natural infection
in an animal in a herd of cattle 100 m away from swine. Were
the circumstances concerning that clinical case indicative of
respiratory infection? If this is not the case then you
cannot conclude anything about airborne transmission.   I
remember one case in a herd where there were no swine at all.
The virus was isolated from the vagina of that particular cow
and was most probably transferred by the veterinarian.

G. Wittmann   The report about the transmission over 100 m was
from a field veterinarian.

V. Bitsch   And you don't know whether that particular animal
showed anterior localisation of pruritus or posterior localisation of pruritus? That is important because anterior
localisation of pruritus is indicative of respiratory infection.
I do not want to question that the virus can be transmitted
over a short distance as an airborne infection but in that
particular case you cannot conclude anything unless you have
the information.

G. Wittmann   I only have the information that the veterinarian
gave me on that particular case. However, in general terms,
if virus up to 10^8 is excreted by pigs, and there is a ventilator in the pig stable blowing out the air to a neighbouring
cattle stable, then it is possible that the cattle will be
infected by this airstream.

V. Bitsch   Yes; we will return to that subject tomorrow. I
think you would agree that one should be careful about making
conclusions from experimental cases in relation to natural
cases. Concerning the transmission of infection from one herd
of cattle to another, the main point is that cattle are not
easily infected, so that even if cattle excrete virus (and

there is ample evidence of that) the infection is not likely
to be caught by a cow next to the infected animal.

G. Wittmann   The same applies to pigs; a pig can remain
healthy even though the animal next to it is infected.

V. Bitsch   Yes, but we have to realise that pigs are more
easily infected by ADV than cattle.   That is easily demonstrated.

G. Wittmann   Yes, but you cannot exclude the possibility of
infection from cattle to cattle.

V. Bitsch   I agree with you; under extreme conditions it
might happen.

P.W. de Leeuw   *(Netherlands)*   I have a few comments on this
subject since we have done some work with cattle in the past.
First of all, there is a strain difference.   We carried out
LD_{50} experiments in cattle - a considerable number - and we
found that with the Northern Ireland 3 strain we needed about
$10^{2.5}$, which is possibly 300 plaque forming units, (pfu),
to infect a one and a half year old steer.   With a moderately
virulent strain for pigs we found that we needed at least tenfold more virus to get the infection started in steers.   We
also checked the virus excretion of these one and a half year
old animals which is approximately the age category in which
you found virus excretion.   In the first lot of animals we
checked oral and pharyngeal fluid and nasal swabs.   In fact
we hardly ever found virus excretion, only occasionally in
animals after they showed the first clinical signs.   If you
slaughter the animals, which we did later, you may find virus
in the mucosa.   We did not find any virus in the secretions.
So I think there are clearly strain differences here.

We have also infected cattle and left other cattle
standing right beside them.   We never observed that one cow
passed the disease to its neighbour.   Of course, that is not
conclusive because in practice there are many more animals but
under these experimental conditions we have not transferred

infection from one cow to the other. I think Dr. Biront may be talking about this in his paper; maybe he has checked on provirus excretion too.

P. Biront *(Belgium)* In vaccination trials when we have infected a cow with ADV we have never observed that it passed to another cow that was not vaccinated.

H. Ludwig Professor Wittmann mentioned that there might be age dependency of infectability of animals. I don't think that has ever really been investigated but it would explain why an adult cow is not easily infected by another cow which is shedding the virus. In other herpes systems the young animals are very vulnerable. I always thought that ADV would be highly virulent for any cattle.

V. Bitsch We have examined quite a lot of isolates from cattle and we have concluded that, practically speaking, only syncytia-forming strains of the virus are capable of infecting cattle by the respiratory route. We will return to that tomorrow.

A. Baskerville That is very interesting; have you any observations on this, Dr. McFerran?

J.B. McFerran We certainly could not support that observation from our strains. All the strains of ADV that we have tried will infect cattle by the intra-nasal route.

V. Bitsch Yes, all strains of ADV are capable of infecting cattle by the respiratory route - in experiments. However, when you test the isolates from natural cases you find that the strains that are highly pathogenic for cattle are the syncytia-forming strains. Only in rare cases will you isolate non-syncytia forming strains from the respiratory tracts of cattle.

J.B. McFerran   This depends on a number of things. You said
'the highly pathogenic strains' - does this mean that you have
strains which have a low pathogenicity for cattle?

V. Bitsch   No. When I mentioned 'highly pathogenic for
cattle' I was referring to strains that will kill a lot of
cattle, or a number of cattle, when you have outbreaks. It is
such strains that are associated with anterior pruritus. In
most such cases we can isolate virus from mucous membranes of
the respiratory tract; in some cases we have even been able to
isolate the virus from lungs of animals. In such cases the
animals showed pruritus on the chest.

J.B McFerran   This is possibly where we differ, because I have
never seen an outbreak of the disease in cattle. I have only
ever seen single cases; once or twice we have seen two animals
involved. This again may be due to strain differences or to
the method of keeping cattle. This is a very vital point
which we will have to talk about.

V. Bitsch   I agree with you and Dr. de Leeuw; we have definitely concluded that there are strain differences with respect
to the ability of the strains to infect cattle by the respiratory route.

H. Ludwig   I believe that syncytia formation is a very
important marker in AD. It reminds me of the situation which
pertains to the study of influenza at present. Those workers
have shown that if there is a cleavage of a certain protein by
trypsin or protease, and this fusion factor is active, then
the virus is virulent; if it is not cleaved it is not virulent
and it does not fuse. So, in that context, I would like to
ask Dr. Dalsgaard a question. Obviously, you have used
syncytia-forming strains to make the antigen and then the
antibody, cutting out the line which is neutralising. Did
you test whether that antibody is fusion inhibiting?

K. Dalsgaard   Unfortunately, no, we have not done that yet.
At the time we did these experiments we were not aware of the
importance of the fusion phenomenon. However, we still have
some of the antibody and I expect Dr. Bitsch will want to test
it for anti-fusion properties. It is a good suggestion.

H. Ludwig   When I was in Giessen, for years we favoured the
theory that the fusion factor in AD might be a non-virion
protein from cells. That idea came from studies where we were
able to inhibit fusion by convalescent sera but we could not
inhibit fusion of infected cells by using antibodies from
hyperimmunised animals which had been treated with inactivated
virus. So it was an indirect conclusion and it would be somewhat in contrast to the herpes simplex system where the fusion
protein seems to be a major glycoprotein belonging to the
virus. The question seems still not to be solved for AD.

B. Liess   (Federal Republic of Germany)   I made an observation some
time ago and we talked about this in culture. Under BUDR the
fused cells got bigger and bigger, far bigger than in the
control cultures which had not been treated with BUDR. I have
no explanation for this as yet but perhaps you can offer one,
particularly in relation to the cell product if, as you say,
there is a fusion factor.

H. Ludwig   I cannot connect it with BUDR. There are a lot
of interconnecting factors.

A. Baskerville   I would like to make one final point about
ADCC in case anyone has the wrong impression. Obviously, it
is more sensitive viewed grossly, but it may be that it is not
measuring the same antibody. We are not in a position to
claim that ADCC is measuring more sensitively the same antibody
that neutralisation is measuring; it may well be that it
measures a totally different antibody. At the moment we have
no way of investigating that.

SESSION IV

VACCINATION

Chairman: P.W. de Leeuw

VACCINATION OF CATTLE AGAINST AUJESZKY'S DISEASE WITH HOMOLOGOUS (HERPES SUIS) AND HETEROLOGOUS (HERPES BOVIS I) VIRUS

P. Biront[1], J. Vandeputte[2], M.B. Pensaert[2] and J. Leunen[1].

[1] Nationaal Instituut voor Diergeneeskundig Onderzoek
Groeselenberg 99, 1180 Brussels, Belgium.

[2] Laboratorium voor Virologie
Fakulteit van de Diergeneeskunde van de Rijksuniversiteit Gent,
Casinoplein 24, 9000 Gent, Belgium.

ABSTRACT

A study was made to examine whether vaccination of cattle against Aujeszky's disease (AD) affords protection upon subsequent intranasal challenge exposure with virulent virus. Vaccinations were performed either subcutaneously with a commercially available oil adjuvanted AD vaccine, in some cases supplemented with Al(OH3), or intranasally with the attenuated NIA-4 strain of Aujeszky's disease virus (ADV) or intranasally with a commercially available TS mutant of BHV-1 (IBR virus). Challenge exposure was performed intranasally with $10^5 LD_{50}$ of the virulent AD virus. In preceding experiments, it had been found that $10^{4.6} TCID_{50}$ of this virulent AD virus strain in primary pig kidney cells represented about 1 LD_{50} for cattle. This LD_{50} was practically the same for cattle with or without antibodies against ADV prior to inoculation. In the seropositive animals, antibodies were present presumably as a consequence of a previous BHV-1 infection in the field.

Intranasal vaccination with NIA-4 or IBR virus did not result in serologic response or protection against challenge exposure. The inactivated vaccine induced a good serologic reaction but the protection upon challenge exposure was very poor. Generalised vaccination of cattle at risk with the inactivated vaccine studied cannot be advised.

In the present experiments, initiation of infection with virulent ADV in cattle always resulted in disease and death.

INTRODUCTION

It was the purpose of the present study to examine whether cattle can be protected by vaccination with an inactivated vaccine against a subsequent intranasal challenge with virulent Aujeszky's disease virus (ADV).

In order to determine the quantity of virulent ADV to be applied for intranasal challenge in cattle, the relationship between the tissue culture infectious dose ($TCID_{50}$) and the lethal dose (LD_{50}) was examined.

Since BHV-1 infection in cattle can result in the formation of neutralising antibodies against ADV (Aquilar-Setien et al., 1979) a study was also made of whether the LD_{50} of ADV in cattle was higher in animals that were seropositive, presumably after IBR infection, than in animals that were seronegative. Furthermore, to find out if a possible cross protective effect could be obtained, a commercially available IBR vaccine was included in the present study.

METHODS

Relationship between $TCID_{50}$ and LD_{50} for ADV in cattle

Twenty cattle were used for determining the LD_{50}. They were divided into 3 groups. In each group there were animals with and without antibodies against ADV.

The three groups received 10^2, 10^3 and 10^4 $TCID_{50}$ virulent ADV intranasally. The challenge strain used was isolated from the lung of a fattening pig that died from AD (Andries et al., 1978).

The animals were examined for clinical signs during the 3 weeks following inoculation. After that time they were also examined for the presence of seroneutralisation antibodies, according to methods described earlier (Andries et al., 1978).

They were subsequently redivided into three groups which then received respectively 10^5, 10^6, 10^7 $TCID_{50}$. One animal not used in the first titration was included in the last trial. Three animals used for the first trial were slaughtered for reasons other than Aujeszky's disease. For virus isolation a 20% suspension of the brain stem was made in phosphate buffered saline. Blind serial passages (PPK cells) were not made.

Vaccination trials

Twenty eight cattle were used for the vaccination as seen in Table 1. The first challenge took place 3 weeks after the last vaccination. Each animal received 10^3 LD_{50} in 10 ml volume (5 ml per nostril). Three weeks after the first challenge the surviving animals received a second challenge intranasally. We examined SN antibodies 3 weeks after each vaccination, 3 weeks after the first challenge and at the time when the animals died or were slaughtered.

TABLE 1

VACCINATION OF CATTLE AGAINST ADV

	Number of animals	Sero-negative prior to vaccination	Sero-positive prior to vaccination	Vaccine	Application
Group 1	12	9	3	Inactivated + oil adjuvants [1]	2 x 5 ml SC
Group 2	6	6	0	Inactivated + oil adjuvants + Al(OH)$_3$	1 x 5 ml + 5 ml AL(OH)$_3$ SC
Group 3	4	1	3	NIA-4-strain	2 x intranasal
Group 4	6	6	0	TS mutant BHV$_1$ [2]	1 x intranasal

[1] Geskyvac Roger Bellon - Neuilly-sur-Seine, France.
[2] Tracherhine Smith Kline - RIT - Rixensart, Genval, Belgium.

The SN antibodies titre against IBR was performed according to the method described by Bitsch, 1978.

The NIA-4 strain and the IBR vaccine contained respectively 10^7 TCID$_{50}$ and $10^{5.7}$ TCID$_{50}$ per dose.

RESULTS

Relationship between TCID$_{50}$ and LD$_{50}$ for ADV in cattle

Reed and Muench calculation revealed that one LD$_{50}$ correlated with $10^{4.2}$ TCID$_{50}$ in the animals that were negative for ADV antibodies and with $10^{5.0}$ TCID$_{50}$ in the seropositive animals. On average, one LD$_{50}$ for both groups correlated with $10^{4.6}$ TCID$_{50}$. The clinical signs observed by these animals were: an incubation period of 6 to 7 days, nervous symptoms such as tremor, ataxia, excitability but no pruritus. Death followed a few hours after the appearance of the first symptoms with a maximum of 12 hours. Virus isolation in the brain stem was positive for all animals that died. None of these animals had built up SN antibodies after challenge with ADV.

TABLE 2

RELATIONSHIP BETWEEN $TCID_{50}$ AND LD_{50} FOR VIRULENT ADV IN CATTLE

Inoculation dose $(TCID)_{50}$[1]	Number of animals that died/total inoculated	
	Seronegative at inoculation	Seropositive at inoculation[2]
10^2	0/4	0/4
10^3	0/4	0/4
10^4	0/2	0/2
10^5	3/5	2/3
10^6	4/4	2/3
10^7	1/1	2/2

[1] Titrated in primary pig kidney cells
[2] Antibodies against ADV presumably due to a previous infection with BHV-1.

Vaccination trials

Table 3 shows the results of the first and second challenge on vaccinated cattle.

The antibody titres of these animals are given in Table 4. The animals vaccinated with the attenuated IBR vaccine had built up a geometric mean homologous SN-titre of 8. Challenge did not result in seroconversion or booster reaction against ADV.

TABLE 3

INTRANASAL CHALLENGE EXPOSURE TO VIRULENT ADV, 3 WEEKS AFTER VACCINATION

Group number	Number of cattle died / total challenged			
	Seronegative at vaccination		Seropositive at vaccination	
	1st challenge	2nd challenge	1st challenge	2nd challenge
1	5/9	1/4	·1/3	0/2
2	3/6	3/3	-	-
3	1/1	-	2/3	1/1
4	6/6	-	-	-

Virus was isolated from the brain stem of all animals except the five that had survived the second challenge. Unfortunately these five animals had to be slaughtered for

SEROLOGIC RESPONSE OF CATTLE PRIOR TO AND AFTER VACCINATION AGAINST ADV

Group number	Vaccine	GMT[1] against ADV (range)			GMT against ADV (range)		
		Prior to vaccination	3 weeks after 1st vaccination	3 weeks after 2nd vaccination	Prior to vaccination	3 weeks after 1st vaccination	3 weeks after 2nd vaccination
1	Inactivated	< 2	21.1(3-48)	128(96-385)	4.9(3-12)	137.2(64-512)	222.8(128-512)
2	Inactivated + Al (OH)$_3$	< 2	33.8(8-384)	-	-	-	-
3	Attenuated NIA-4	< 2	NT	NT	12(6-24)	13.9(6-32)	17.1(12-32)
4	TS mutant BHV-1	< 2	1.2(<2-2)	-	-	-	-

[1] GMT: geometric mean SN-titre.

practical reasons 8 days after the second challenge. This is important to mention because in some vaccinated animals that showed symptoms upon the second challenge exposure, the incubation period lasted as long as 8 to 12 days.

The clinical signs observed were the same as described in the LD_{50} experiment.

CONCLUSIONS

1. The minimal infectious dose for cattle with or without ADV antibodies (cross reaction IBR infection) was practically the same ($10^{4.6} \longleftrightarrow 10^5$ $TCID_{50}$).
2. Vaccination with IBR vaccine gives no protection against ADV.
3. No surviving animal showed an increase in SN titre against ADV after challenge exposure.
   Once an infection with ADV has started in cattle, clinical signs will appear and the disease will run a fatal course.
4. Only vaccination with the inactivated vaccine caused a clearcut serologic response.
   The protection rate was still very poor.
5. It remains unexplained why some animals did not become sick after a first challenge exposure while death occurred after the second challenge. Such a result was unexpected considering that the dose was 10^3 LD_{50}.

REFERENCES

Andries, K., Pensaert, M.B. and Vandeputte, J., 1978. Effect of experimental infection with pseudorabies virus on pigs with maternal immunity from vaccinated sows. Am. J. Vet. Res., 39, 1282-1285.
Aquilar-Setien, R., Vandeputte, J. and Pastoret, P.P., 1979. Présence concommittante chez les bovins et les porcs d'anticorps neutralisant le virus de la rhinotrachéite infectieuse bovine et celui de la maladie d'Aujeszky après contact avec le virus homologue. Ann. Med. Vét. 123, 275-285.
Bitsch, V., 1978. The P_{24} modification of the infectious bovine rhinotracheitis virus seroneutralisation test. Acta. Vet. Scand. 19, 497-505.

IMMUNOPROPHYLAXIS OF AUJESZKY'S DISEASE IN ITALY

T. Frescura[1], D. Cessi[2], P. Vivoli[1] and F. De Simone[2]

[1] Istituto Zooprofilattico Sperimentale
dell'Umbria e delle Marche
06100 Perugia, Italy.
[2] Istituto Zooprofilattico Sperimentale
della Lombardia e dell'Emilia
25100 Brescia, Italy.

ABSTRACT

The use of inactivated and attenuated vaccines against Aujeszky's disease in Italy is described.

The inactivated vaccine is successful in preventing the disease in healthy conditions, whereas in strongly infected areas, particularly where there is intensive pig production, the disease is more successfully controlled by the use of the attenuated vaccine.

INTRODUCTION

Aujeszky's disease (AD) in pigs was first recognised in Italy during the fifties. Since that time the disease has increasingly spread among pigs of all ages, but mostly affecting piglets and sows, in which it causes abortions. Although the disease is prevalent all over Italy, it occurs mostly in the north and in the central part of the country, where pig production is concentrated.

According to research carried out in Lombardia and Emilia, where pig production represents 46% of national production, the disease occurs in about 50% of the breeding farms, in 30% of the fattening farms and in 9% of the domestic piggeries. Results obtained in the central part of Italy are not different from the ones apparent in the north. In southern Italy, AD seldom occurs, due to the poor development of pig production. Because of the economic losses from outbreaks of the disease which have become more and more severe and frequent, harmless and adequate vaccines have increasingly been required. Therefore the Istituto Zooprofilattico of Perugia and Brescia have prepared two types of vaccine (inactivated and attenuated live viruses) which have both been experimented on for a long time.

INACTIVATED VACCINE

This vaccine is produced at the Istituto Zooprofilattico

G. Wittmann, S.A. Hall (eds), Aujeszky's Disease. ISBN-13:978-94-009-7555-2

of Perugia. The virus is cultivated on a large scale and with
a high titre infecting BHK cells grown in suspension. The vaccine is prepared by adding Alhydrogel to supernatant infected
fluids followed by formalin inactivation. Saponin is then added.

The potency tests carried out in the laboratory during the
last few years confirm that the injection of the vaccine stim-
ulates the production of neutralising antibodies in most of the
subjects. Pigs vaccinated for the first time show a rather low
antibody titre which rises sharply after the second vaccination.

Challenge showed that resistance to AD is not strictly
correlated with the detectable antibodies; in fact some pigs
without neutralising antibodies appeared to be protected.
Laboratory findings were largely confirmed by results in the
field.

Production of the inactivated vaccine at the Istituto
Zooprofilattico of Perugia began in 1964. Since then the
immunogenicity has been improved and production has increased
to 2 million doses per year.

Preventive vaccination in healthy herds requires two
interventions carried out at an interval of 15 - 30 days. Sows
must be systematically revaccinated 30 days before farrowing in
order to protect piglets during the first weeks of life.
Generally piglets must be vaccinated for the first time during
weaning, namely, when they are 4 weeks old. Pigs must be
systematically revaccinated every 6 months. A 3 ml dose must
be injected subcutaneously in 1 month old piglets, a 5 ml dose
is used in older pigs.

ATTENUATED LIVE VACCINE

The virus for the production of this vaccine is the
Rumanian strain BUK received after 210 passages in chicken
embryos and further attenuated in the laboratories of the
Istituto Zooprofilattico of Brescia by 206 passages in chick
embryo fibroblast cell cultures. The virus is grown on chicken
fibroblasts in rolling bottles. It is gathered after 24 hours'
incubation and lyophilised. The fluid used to reconstitute
the lyophilised virus contains Alhydrogel. The safety test has

been carried out by serial back-passages on piglets without antibodies and by vaccinating pregnant sows.

Potency tests were performed measuring the neutralising antibodies. The live attenuated vaccine has been produced in the Istituto Zooprofilattico of Brescia since 1968 and the yearly production has been steadily increasing to the present level of 5 million doses per year. The vaccine is used in infected herds or in threatened ones. Animals of every age can be vaccinated. A 1 ml dose must be injected subcutaneously regardless of the age and weight of the pig.

CONCLUSIONS

Prevention or control of AD cannot be achieved by sanitary and hygienic measures, particularly in intensive herds; only an active immunisation programme can prevent the economic losses due to the disease. The different conditions of production and environment, and the high incidence of the disease in Italy, provide a strong justification for the use of the two kinds of vaccines.

In practice, the inactivated vaccine is used for the prophylaxis of the disease in healthy piggeries and farms, whilst the live attenuated vaccine is necessary in infected or threatened piggeries.

From our experience we can confidently say that the use of these vaccines enables us to limit, as far as possible, the economic losses caused by Aujeszky's disease.

COMPARISON OF INTRANASAL AND PARENTERAL VACCINATION AGAINST AUJESZKY'S DISEASE IN 12-WEEK-OLD PIGS FROM IMMUNISED DAMS

P.W. de Leeuw[1], J.M. Wijsmuller[2], J.W. Zantinga[3] and M.J.M. Tielen[4]

[1]Central Veterinary Institute, Department of Virology, 39 Houtribweg, 8221 RA Lelystad,

[2]Veterinary Practice Hintham, 5246 AM Rosmalen,

[3]Duphar B.V, P.O. Box 2, 1380 AA Weesp,

[4]Regional Animal Health Service Noord-Brabant, Molenwijkseweg 48, 5282 SC Boxtel, The Netherlands.

ABSTRACT

A pilot experiment in groups of five 10-week-old seronegative pigs showed that intranasal (i.n.) vaccination with Bartha's K strain of Aujeszky's disease (AD) virus induced a good antibody response and resulted in nearly complete protection against disease following severe i.n. challenge two months post-vaccination (p.v.). In addition, excretion of challenge virus was much reduced as compared to that of controls. There was little difference in these respects between pigs vaccinated with 10^4, 10^6 or 10^8 plaque forming units. No untoward reactions following i.n. vaccination were observed.

The main experiment was done with 12-week-old pigs from dams revaccinated shortly before parturition. All pigs had maternal antibodies detectable in a sensitive neutralisation test. They were randomly distributed in three groups of ten and one of nine. One group was vaccinated intranasally with 10^6 TCID$_{50}$ of the Bartha strain, two groups parenterally with a commercially available modified live virus vaccine based on the same strain and one group was left unvaccinated. After three weeks one of the parenterally vaccinated groups was revaccinated.

Intramuscular (i.m.) vaccination had a slow but distinct serologic effect; a second i.m. vaccination after three weeks resulted in a booster response. I.n. vaccination gave a faster serologic effect than i.m. vaccination while titres continued to increase over a long period.

Six pigs of each group were challenged after 6 weeks and four pigs after 4 months, together with four or five unvaccinated controls.

At 6 weeks p.v., one of the control pigs died after challenge and the others showed a mean growth arrest period of 12 days, reflecting severe clinical disease. No vaccinated pigs died. The animals vaccinated once intramuscularly were less severely affected than the controls, the mean growth arrest period being 6.5 days. Pigs vaccinated intranasally or twice intramuscularly were very well protected and on an average did not lose weight.

At 4 months p.v., all pigs survived the challenge, but clinical disease of varying severity developed in all groups. Intranasally vaccinated pigs were markedly better protected than pigs vaccinated twice intramuscularly, despite the fact that the latter had somewhat higher serum antibody titres. The mean growth arrest periods of the different groups were more than 19 days for the controls, 13.5 and 12 days for pigs vaccinated intramuscularly once or twice and 6.5 days for intranasally vaccinated pigs.

G. Wittmann, S.A. Hall (eds), Aujeszky's Disease. ISBN-13:978-94-009-7555-2

*Particularly after challenge at 6 weeks p.v., the intranasally vac-
cinated pigs excreted much less virus than the parenterally vaccinated pigs.
In this respect there was little difference between pigs vaccinated intramuscularly once or twice, but both categories excreted less virus than the
controls. A similar pattern, though less marked, was observed after challenge at 4 months p.v.*

*It is concluded that i.n. vaccination of pigs against AD is promising
enough to warrant further study, particularly as a means to overcome interference of maternal antibodies with active immunisation.*

INTRODUCTION

One of the major problems in protecting a swine population
against Aujeszky's disease (AD) by vaccination, is to achieve
active immunisation of pigs from immunised dams. It is a
particularly difficult problem if such pigs are vaccinated at a
relatively young age when the effect of parenteral vaccination
will be less than in seronegative pigs (Tielen et al., 1980).
When the pigs grow older, i.e. when maternal antibody titres
decrease and more and more animals become seronegative, better
overall results of a vaccination may be expected. The
epizootiological situation, however, may call for vaccination
as early as possible. Under such conditions the optimum moment
to vaccinate is difficult to determine, as it is influenced by
many variables, among which are the vaccine(s) and the vaccination scheme(s) used. Fattening herds may pose a special problem as the pigs may originate from different breeders using
different prophylactic measures against AD.

Intranasal (i.n.) vaccination against AD of pigs from
immunised dams has not been studied, to our knowledge, although
encouraging results were obtained in seronegative pigs (McFerran
and Dow, 1975). Yet this approach appears logical in view of
the pathogenesis of the disease and because one may expect that
maternal antibodies will not interfere to the same extent as
they appear to do in the case of parenteral vaccination (Tielen
et al., 1980).

In this report the results of experiments on i.n. vaccination of pigs are recorded and compared with those obtained
after parenteral vaccination according to a scheme that appeared
to give satisfactory results in the field (Wijsmuller, 1980).

MATERIALS AND METHODS

Experimental animals

Seronegative pigs were from the Dutch Landrace minimal disease (MD) herd of the Central Veterinary Institute, in which AD has never occurred. The other pigs were cross-breds from a privately owned herd, where clinical AD had not been observed in recent years.

Vaccination and challenge

Intramuscular (i.m.) vaccination was done with Duvaxyn-Aujeszky[1] a modified live virus vaccine based on Bartha's K strain of Aujeszky's disease virus (ADV), using the recommended dose (2 ml). The titre of this vaccine is 10^5 tissue culture infective doses fifty ($TCID_{50}$) per ml. For i.n. vaccination the same virus strain, multiplied in pig kidney cells, was used. The vaccination was performed by instilling 0.5 ml of the· vaccine virus suspension drop by drop into each nostril, while holding the head of the pig slightly backwards.

Challenge with virulent ADV was carried out intranasally using the technique employed for the i.n. vaccination. The virus used was the Northern Ireland Aujeszky Three (NIA-3) strain (McFerran and Dow, 1975; kindly provided by Dr. J.B. McFerran, Stormont, Belfast, Northern Ireland), passaged six times in secondary pig kidney (PK_2) cell cultures. The challenge dose was 10^5 plaque forming units (p.f.u.) in PK_2 cell cultures as described earlier (De Leeuw and Tiessink, 1980).

Before i.n. vaccination and challenge, the pigs were given a tranquilliser[2].

Sampling procedures, virus titration and neutralisation test

Blood samples were taken from the jugular vein. Neutralising antibodies in sera were titrated in a microtitre system, using PK_2 cells and a serum/virus incubation period of 24 h at 37^oC to obtain high sensitivity (Bitsch and Eskildsen, 1976).

[1]Produced by Duphar, B.V., Weesp, the Netherlands.
[2]Stresnil, Janssen Pharmaceutica, Beerse, Belgium.

Sera were diluted in duplicate in two-fold steps and mixed with equal volumes (0.05 ml) of a NIA-3 virus suspension, containing approximately 200 $TCID_{50}$ to allow for thermo-inactivation during the incubation period. After 24 h at 37°C, on average 30-100 $TCID_{50}/0.05$ ml were recovered from control virus suspensions, i.e. sera were tested against 30-100 $TCID_{50}$. Serum antibody titres were determined by the 50% endpoint method of Reed and Muench; they are given as log_{10} values.

Oro-pharyngeal (OP) fluid samples were collected, treated and assayed for virus as described (De Leeuw et al., 1979), but 4 ml of buffer was added to the swabs and arctone extraction was omitted. Virus titres are expressed as the number of p.f.u./ ml in PK_2 cell cultures.

Experiments

Experiment 1. Twenty seronegative pigs from three sows in the MD herd were randomly distributed in four groups of five and each group was housed in an isolation room. At the age of 10 weeks three groups were intranasally vaccinated with 10^4, 10^6 or 10^8 p.f.u. respectively. The fourth group served as a control. All pigs were weighed once a week until the day after challenge and then three times weekly. Challenge was made two months p.v. Blood samples were taken weekly; OP swabs daily for ten days after vaccination and after challenge.

Experiment 2. Three gilts and three sows in a private herd, where vaccination against AD was done with Duvaxyn-Aujeszky every six months, received their revaccination 4 - 5 weeks before parturition. To check for wild virus infections, seven piglets of the MD herd were obtained and distributed over the six litters designated for the experiment. These control pigs were of the same age as their new litter mates; they were transferred when three to five days old. All 46 pigs were weaned at the age of 5 weeks and 2 weeks later transported to the experimental farm of Duphar. Here they were randomly distributed in groups of nine or ten. Vaccination was done at the age of 12 weeks. Two groups were vaccinated intramuscularly, one group intra-nasally and one group remained unvaccinated. The pigs from the

MD herd also remained unvaccinated. For i.n. vaccination a
virus suspension containing 10^6 TCID$_{50}$/ml (produced and titrated
by Duphar) was used. The intranasally vaccinated pigs were
housed in the same (open) building, but at some distance from
the other pigs, including the pigs from the MD herd. After
three weeks one of the intramuscularly vaccinated groups was
revaccinated in the same manner. A first challenge was carried
out 6 weeks after (the first) vaccination with groups of six
vaccinated pigs and five controls; the remainder was challenged
four months p.v. The seven control pigs from the MD herd were
not challenged. Both challenges were performed in the isolation
units of the Central Veterinary Institute at Lelystad. Weighing
was done as in Experiment 1, blood samples were taken regularly
though less frequently than in the first experiment and OP swabs
were obtained only after challenge.

RESULTS

   We are reporting only the most important results, referring
for further details to the original paper (in preparation).

Experiment 1

   No untoward reactions were observed after i.n. vaccination
with the three doses used although the average body temperatures
of pigs in two of the three vaccinated groups (the 10^4 and 10^8
groups) were higher than usual (40 to 40.2°C instead of 39.8°C)
for three to four days p.v. The mean weight curves of the
groups of vaccinated pigs and the curve of the control pigs ran
parallel until the time of challenge.

   At least two virus positive OP fluid samples were obtained
from each vaccinated pig during the first ten days p.v. On
average, virus excretion in the 10^8 group started earlier and
reached somewhat higher levels than in the other two groups.
The highest titres found were $10^{4.7}$, $10^{3.6}$ and $10^{5.4}$ p.f.u./ml
of OP fluid in the 10^4, 10^6 and 10^8 groups, respectively.

   The mean serological responses of the different groups
showed little variation. The mean serum antibody titre of pigs
in the 10^8 group was considerably higher at one week p.v. than

that of pigs in the other groups but thereafter the curves
were very similar and at the time of challenge the mean titres
of the different vaccinated groups were nearly the same (Table 1).

TABLE 1

SUMMARISED RESULTS OF EXPERIMENT 1, INTRANASAL VACCINATION OF SERONEGATIVE
PIGS

Vaccination dose[1] (p.f.u.)	Number of pigs	Mean serum titre[2] two months p.v. ($\log_{10}$)	Protection against challenge[3]	
			Number that died	Mean growth arrest period survivors (days)
10^4	5	1.7	−	2.5
10^6	5	1.5	−	2.5
10^8	5	1.6	−	−
−	5	−	1	13.0

[1]Pigs aged 10 weeks vaccinated with Bartha's K strain of ADV, 0.5 ml into
each nostril.

[2]Titres determined in a microtitre neutralising test with an incubation
period of the serum/virus mixture of 24 h at 37°C.

[3]Challenged intranasally with 10^5 p.f.u. of the NIA-3 strain of ADV two
months p.v.

Three days after challenge, all five control pigs had
fever, were reluctant to move and to eat and vomited. One of
them died on the fifth day. The other four all had the
characteristic hoarse squeal when handled, developed severe
rhinitis which eventually became purulent and two showed signs
of central nervous system disturbances. The animals started to
recover on days 8 to 10. In contrast, symptoms in the vaccinated pigs, if present, were mild and did not last long. Usually
the only symptoms were fever and a reduced appetite. Clinically
there was no clear-cut difference between the 10^4, 10^6 and the
10^8 groups. The disease pattern described above, can be recorded in a more objective manner by the use of weight curves
(Figure 1). Whereas the controls that survived lost on average
5.5 kg and needed 13 days to regain the weight they had at the
time of challenge (period of growth arrest), the weight curves
of the groups of vaccinated pigs showed little or no depression.
The curves also show that the two to three days of growth arrest

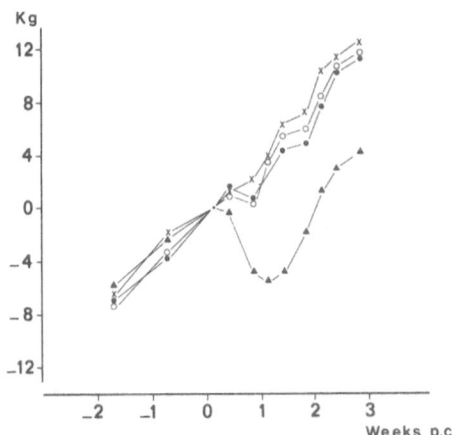

Fig. 1. Mean weight curves of groups of five intranasally vaccinated
pigs before and after challenge. Seronegative pigs were vaccinated at the age of 10 weeks; they were intranasally challenged after
2 months. ● Vaccinated with 10^4 p.f.u. of the Bartha strain of
ADV, o with 10^6 p.f.u. and x with 10^8 p.f.u.; ▲ were non-vaccinated controls (mean of four, one died).

observed in the 10^4 and 10^6 groups were compensated quickly
as there appears to be no significant effect on the expected
course of the curves.

Average virus excretion after challenge of intranasally
vaccinated pigs was considerably less than that observed in the
controls. Here again, the differences between the 10^4, 10^6 and
10^8 groups appeared insignificant.

Experiment 2

All seven sentinel pigs from the MD herd remained serologically negative for ADV antibodies throughout the experiment.

No untoward reactions or body temperature increases were
observed in any of the vaccinated pigs. Growth rates of the
different groups were comparable until the time of challenge.

The mean serological responses after vaccination of pigs
challenged in the first part of the experiment are shown in
Figure 2. Intramuscular vaccination resulted first in a change
in the slope of the curve and was later followed by an increase
in the mean titre. The second i.m. vaccination produced a
booster response in nearly all pigs. After i.n. vaccination

150

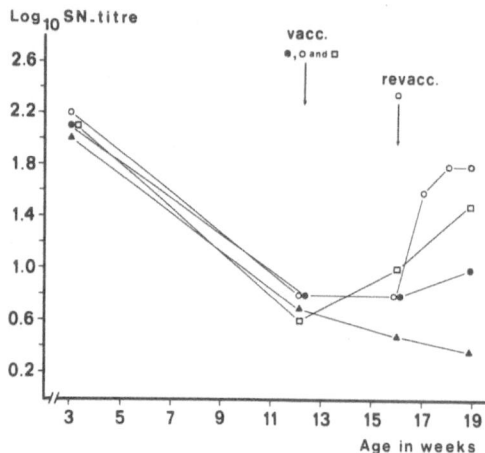

Fig. 2. Mean serological responses of groups of six pigs from immunised
dams after vaccination at the age of 12 weeks. ● once and o twice
vaccinated intramuscularly with a modified live virus vaccine
based on the Bartha strain,□ vaccinated intranasally once with
10^6 TCID50 of the same strain, ▲ non-vaccinated controls.

the mean titre showed a continuous increase over the six weeks
observation period (Figure 2).

Judging from clinical signs, the intranasally vaccinated
pigs appeared to be the best protected of the groups challenged
six weeks p.v. The group vaccinated twice intramuscularly also
appeared to be protected very well. In the intranasally
vaccinated group the mean body temperatures remained below 40°C
after challenge, whereas in the twice intramuscularly vaccinated
group average temperatures of ≥ 40°C were recorded on three
consecutive days. The group of pigs vaccinated intramuscularly
once was clearly less well protected than the two groups
mentioned above, but better protected than the controls. Of
this last group one animal died on day seven; the vaccinated
pigs all survived the challenge. This clinical picture was
largely reflected by the weight curves and the mean growth
arrest periods derived thereof (Table 2). However, the difference in clinical signs between the group vaccinated intranasally
and that vaccinated twice intramuscularly does not show. In
fact the growth curves of both groups were barely affected by the
challenge.

TABLE 2

SUMMARISED RESULTS OF EXPERIMENT 2, COMPARISON OF VACCINATION ROUTES AND
REGIMENS IN 12-WEEK-OLD PIGS FROM IMMUNISED DAMS

Number of pigs	Mean serum titre when vaccinated ($\log_{10}$)	Vacci-nation[1]	Chall-enged after	Mean titre when chall-enged ($\log_{10}$)	Mean growth arrest period after challenge (days)
6	0.8	i.m. 1x		1.0	7
6	0.8	i.m. 2x	6	1.8	-
6	0.6	i.n.	weeks	1.5	-
5	0.7	-		0.4	12[2]
4	0.8	i.m. 1x		1.4	13.5
4	0.8	i.m. 2x	4	2.0	12
4	0.7	i.n.	months	1.9	6.5
4	1.0	-		-	>19[3]

[1]Intramuscular (i.m.) vaccination was done with Duvaxyn-Aujeszky (Duphar
B.V., Weesp, the Netherlands) once (1x) or twice (2x) with three weeks in
between; intranasal (i.n.) vaccination with a virus suspension having a
titre of 10^6 TCID50.

[2]Average of four; one pig died after the challenge. All other pigs in this
experiment survived the challenge.

[3]Observations terminated 19 days post challenge. For further explanation,
see Table 1 and text.

Excretion of challenge virus in intramuscularly vaccinated
pigs was less than that in control pigs, particularly with
respect to the number of days virus was excreted, but there was
little difference between the groups that had been vaccinated
once or twice. The mean virus titre in OP fluid of intranasally
vaccinated pigs was far less than that in any of the other
groups (Figure 3).

The mean serum antibody titres of groups of pigs challenged
in the second part of Experiment 2, initially followed the same
pattern as shown on Figure 2. Between six weeks and four months
p.v., the mean titres of the groups vaccinated intranasally
and once intramuscularly continued to rise. At the time of
challenge the average titres of the pigs vaccinated intranasally
and those vaccinated twice intramuscularly were nearly the same
(Table 2).

All vaccinated and control pigs survived the challenge,
but clinically there were marked differences between the groups

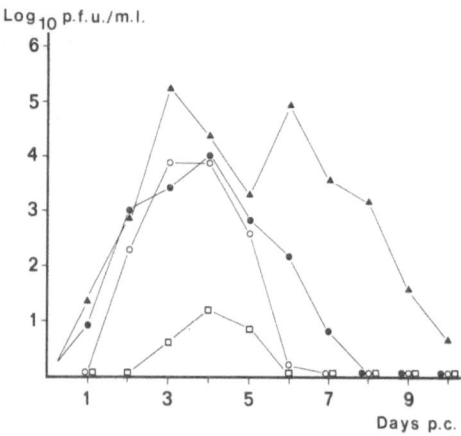

Fig. 3. Mean virus titres of oropharyngeal fluid samples of vaccinated
pigs from immunised dams after challenge six weeks p.v. Symbols
used are the same in Figure 2; four pigs in each group were
sampled.

as illustrated by the mean growth arrest periods shown on
Table 2. In contrast to the first challenge six weeks p.v.,
however, there was little difference in the degree of protection
between the two intramuscularly vaccinated groups. The intranasally vaccinated pigs clearly performed better than the
parenterally vaccinated pigs, including those that had been
vaccinated twice.

Virus excretion after challenge on an average was less
in vaccinated than in control pigs, both in titre and duration.
However, the differences between vaccinated and control pigs
and between intranasally and intramuscularly vaccinated pigs,
were not as marked as observed after the challenge at six
weeks p.v.

DISCUSSION

Under experimental conditions i.n. installation of virus
in pigs aged 10 to 12 weeks proved quite easy to perform and,
in fact, the use of a tranquilliser was superfluous. No
distinct local or generalised reactions were observed following
i.n. vaccination. In Experiment 1 some of the pigs in the 10^4
and 10^8 groups were febrile for a few days, but their behaviour
and growth performance appeared unaltered.

The results obtained with i.n. vaccination of seronegative pigs (Figure 1, Table 1) were considered highly satisfactory. All three vaccinated groups developed a good serologic response, were well protected against disease following challenge two months p.v. and excreted little virulent virus. Particularly with respect to the last two criteria, the results were better than those obtained under similar conditions with two parenteral vaccinations of an inactivated and a modified live virus vaccine (De Leeuw and Tiessink, 1980). Our results therefore confirm those of McFerran and Dow (1975) who compared i.n. and i.m. vaccination with Bartha's K strain of ADV in seronegative pigs and observed that intranasally vaccinated pigs were better protected and excreted less challenge virus than intramuscularly vaccinated pigs. These authors found little vaccine virus excretion after i.n. vaccination and considered it unlikely that it would be enough to infect other litters. However, in Experiment 1 rather high titres of up to $10^{5.4}$ p.f.u./ml of OP fluid were found, suggesting that spread of vaccine virus may occur. It is obvious that this subject requires further study, both in seronegative pigs and in pigs with maternal antibodies.

Although in Experiment 1 no significant differences were observed in results obtained with vaccine doses of 10^4, 10^6 and 10^8 p.f.u.; it did not appear unlikely that in seropositive pigs the dose used for i.n. vaccination would be more critical. Therefore in the second experiment a dose well above the 10^4 level was used, i.e. 10^6 $TCID_{50}$.

To check for wild virus infections, piglets from the MD herd were placed as sentinels in the litters used in Experiment 2. Since all seven pigs remained serologically negative, one may reasonably assume that no wild virus infections occurred during the experiment. In addition, the intramuscularly vaccinated pigs apparently did not spread the vaccine virus. One cannot draw a similar conclusion with respect to the intranasally vaccinated pigs as they were housed at some distance from the sentinels.

The results obtained with i.n. vaccination of pigs with maternal antibodies were equal to or better than those obtained with parenteral vaccination, even after two i.m. injections

(Table 2). Although at six weeks p.v. both intranasally and twice intramuscularly vaccinated pigs proved to be adequately protected against disease, the intranasally vaccinated pigs excreted considerably less virus after challenge. At four months p.v., this latter difference was less marked, but at this stage the degree of protection turned out to the advantage of intranasally vaccinated pigs (Table 2). Pigs vaccinated intramuscularly once were clearly less well protected than those vaccinated twice when challenged six weeks p.v.; at four months p.v., however, there was remarkably little difference. In addition, virus excretion of the pigs in these groups was very similar. Unvaccinated litter mates in each instance were more severely affected and excreted more virus than vaccinated pigs. From these last results one may conclude that under the conditions of the herd where this experiment was started, a single i.m. vaccination with Duvaxyn-Aujeszky of pigs of about 12 weeks will have a beneficial effect on herd immunity. A second i.m. vaccination after three weeks would only have a temporary effect as far as protection against AD is concerned. The stronger serological response, however, may be of importance for young breeding stock.

Comparison of the mean serum antibody titres of the different groups and the mean growth arrest periods observed after challenge (Table 2), shows that the predictive value of the former as regards protection is limited. The relationship is apparently influenced by the time which has elapsed since the vaccination and by the route of vaccination. This is reasonable as one may assume that i.n. vaccination will result in better local immunity than i.m. vaccination. It probably also explains the striking difference observed in virus excretion after challenge of pigs vaccinated by the i.n. or i.m. route.

In our opinion the results reported here of i.n. vaccination of pigs against AD, are promising enough to warrant further study, despite a possibly more difficult administration of the vaccine.

ACKNOWLEDGEMENTS

The authors wish to thank Mr. J.W.A. Tiessink and Mr. W.A.M. van Rossum for excellent technical assistance and Dr. A.C.A. van Exsel for his help and stimulating interest.

REFERENCES

Bitsch, V. and Eskildsen, M. 1976. A comparative examination of swine sera for antibody to Aujeszky virus with the conventional test and a modified virus-serum neutralization test and a modified direct complement fixation test. Acta Vet. Scand., 17, 142-152.

De Leeuw, P.W., Tiessink, J.W.A. and van Bekkum, J.G. 1979. The challenge of vaccinated pigs with foot-and-mouth disease virus. Zbl. Vet. Med. B, 26, 98-109.

De Leeuw, P.W. and Tiessink, J.W.A. 1980. Evaluation of Aujeszky's disease virus vaccines. Proc. IPVS congress, Copenhagen, p.112.

McFerran, J.B. and Dow, C. 1975. Studies on immunisation of pigs with the Bartha strain of Aujeszky's disease virus. Res. Vet. Sc., 19, 17-22.

Tielen, M.J.M., Brus, D.H.J., van Exsel, A.C.A., Akkermans, J.P.W.M. and Rondhuis, P.R. 1980. Vaccinatie van mestbiggen tegen de ziekte van Aujeszky. Een onderzoek naar de weerstand van mestvarkens na enting met verschillende entstoffen op een leeftijd van 4-9 weken. Tijdschr. Diergeneesk., 105, 826-834.

Wijsmuller, J.M. 1980. De ziekte van Aujeszky: ent-problematiek en ent-advies. Tijdschr. Diergeneesk., 105, 108-110.

ASSESSMENT OF AUJESZKY'S VACCINATION PROGRAMME IN THE REPUBLIC OF IRELAND

P.J. O'Connor and P. Lenihan

Department of Agriculture, Veterinary Research Laboratory,
Abbotstown, Castleknock, Co. Dublin, Ireland.

ABSTRACT

By 1980 the prevalence of clinical Aujeszky's disease (AD) in the Republic of Ireland, together with evidence of widespread subclinical infection, was such that it was agreed to license AD vaccine. Only inactivated vaccines are permitted. The importation and distribution of vaccine are subject to control by the Department of Agriculture in order to maintain surveillance of vaccinated herds. To date 69 breeding herds and 9 fattening herds have been vaccinated with encouraging results. However, careful monitoring of the disease over the next decade should allow a more critical appraisal of its value.

Since 1973, when Aujeszky's disease (AD) was first recognised as causing serious mortality in a large piggery, the disease has steadily increased in importance in the Republic of Ireland. To date the disease has been confirmed in 80 large pig units. The distribution of these units is shown in Figure 1. During 1980 17 new cases were recorded, the greatest in any one year since 1973.

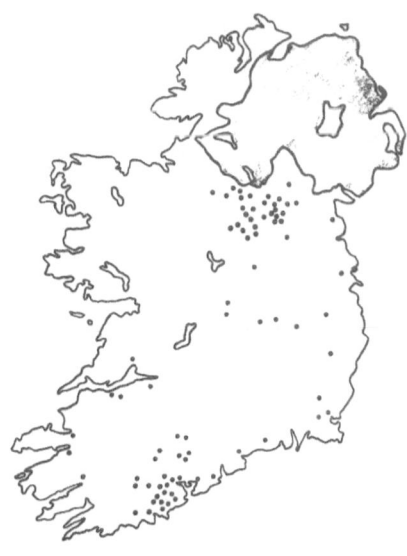

Fig. 1. Distribution of AD infected herds in the Republic of Ireland.

G. Wittmann, S.A. Hall (eds), Aujeszky's Disease. ISBN-13:978-94-009-7555-2

The emergence of AD as a herd problem coincided with the period when radical restructuring was taking place within the pig industry. Many producers had borrowed heavily to finance their enterprises. Their repayments were based on fairly optimistic production targets and any upset such as AD obviously imposed a severe financial burden on those unfortunate enough to suffer disease.

An analysis of the disease in infected breeding herds showed that more than half the cases occurred in herds ranging in size between 100 and 1 700 sows. As these herds accounted for 13% of the national sow population the disease was much more important than the numbers of infected herds would suggest.

The various zoosanitary control measures which were applied proved inadequate to stem the spread of virus within infected herds. Furthermore, as AD was not a notifiable disease, there were no control measures which could prevent the movement of infected carrier stock between farms. Everything pointed to the disease continuing to escalate and by 1979 the disease had become an emotive issue among pig producers who demanded that some action should be taken to control the spread of virus.

The level of clinical disease coupled with evidence of widespread subclinical infection, based on the results of serological surveys, was such that it was deemed impractical at the time to attempt a programme of eradication. An alternative to an eradication policy was to allow vaccine to be used. At this time information from various countries including the Netherlands, France and the USA suggested that vaccine afforded a considerable measure of success in disease control. After much consideration, in 1980 the Department of Agriculture agreed to license AD vaccine subject to certain controls.

By tradition live virus vaccines were not permitted for use in livestock. This was because of the remote risk of introducing, as a contaminant, an exotic virus such as Foot and Mouth or Swine Fever virus. Consequently, the Department of Agriculture decided that only inactivated AD vaccine would be sanctioned for use. Licences are granted provided vaccine is inactivated and the manufacturing plant complies with Department standards. Vaccine must also afford protection under

specified challenge experiments in Abbotstown. Two vaccines
have already been evaluated and found effective (Tables 1 and
2).

TABLE 1

PSEUDORABIES VACCINE (SALSBURY LABORATORIES) - RESULTS 15 DAYS AFTER I.N.
CHALLENGE WITH $10^{6.5}$ $TCID_{50}$ NIA^{-3}

	Died	Survived
Vaccinates	1	14
Controls	9	4

TABLE 2

PSEUDORABIES VACCINE (NORDEN LABORATORIES) - RESULTS 15 DAYS AFTER I.N.
CHALLENGE WITH $10^{6.5}$ $TCID_{50}$ NIA^{-3}

	Died	Survived
Vaccinates	2	14
Controls	12	1

To date only one vaccine has been licensed for use -
Salsbury Pseudorabies Vaccine - and it has been in use since
February 1980. It is recommended for use in sows, and in pigs
of two weeks or older. Pigs should be vaccinated with 2 ml
and breeding stock with 4 ml, with a repeat dose after two
weeks.

The second AD inactivated vaccine - Norden Pseudorabies
Vaccine - should be available shortly. The recommendation for
this vaccine is a single 2 ml injection for all age groups.
This feature should make its administration much simpler.

Following approval of any AD vaccine the importing firm
is required to furnish to the Department of Agriculture monthly
returns of all vaccine imported. Only veterinary surgeons
can be supplied and a list of those receiving vaccine must
also be furnished.

The only restriction imposed by the Department of
Agriculture on those veterinary surgeons who wish to use AD
vaccine is an obligation to furnish details as laid out in
document ADV2 (Figure 2). The reason for controlling vaccine

ADV 2

Name of herd owner: Veterinary Practitioner:

Address: Address:

Date of initial vaccination:_____

Description of Herd:

Breeding & Weaner   Breeding & Fattening   Fattening
   Production

_____   _____   _____

Size of herd:

No. of Sows_____   No. of fatteners_____

Age Group Vaccinated:

Breeding Stock_____   Fatteners_____   Others_____

Reason for Vaccination:

- In Face of Active Disease   _____
- To Control Recurrence of Disease   _____
- For Prophylaxis   _____

Fig. 2. Herd information on use of Aujeszky's Vaccine.

in this fashion is in order to maintain a surveillance of the number of herds and type of pigs which have been vaccinated. Furthermore, it will allow an evaluation of vaccine efficiency.

Data, compiled from ADV2 forms, show that AD vaccine has been used in 69 breeding herds. It can be seen from Table 3 that although vaccine has been used in herds of various sizes a greater proportion of the larger herds has been vaccinated. This is understandable considering the relatively greater economic losses that would be sustained should disease occur.

Breeding herds which have been vaccinated to date can be divided into 3 categories:-

1) Herds suffering clinical disease: 11 such herds have vaccinated all stock in the face of infection.

TABLE 3

ANALYSIS OF VACCINATED BREEDING HERDS - ACCORDING TO SIZE.

Breeding herd size (sows)	50-100	100-200	200-500	500+
Number of herds vaccinated	15	25	15	14
Herds vaccinated %	2.5%	14%	25%	58%

2)   Herds with a previous history of clinical disease:
     17 such herds have used vaccine. All replacement stock
     are vaccinated on entry, but the decision to vaccinate
     the remainder of the breeding stock is based on the results
     of serological surveillance. In herds where high anti-
     body titres can be demonstrated in homebred stock vaccine
     is not administered.

3)   Herds without a history of AD: 41 such herds have been
     vaccinated prophylactically. In these herds vaccine
     is confined to parent stock.

     Approximately 13% of sows are located in herds where
AD has been diagnosed. In the larger herds the virus can be
expected to have become endemic. Consequently transfer of
virus by carrier pigs, between breeding herds and fattening herds,
must occur. However, as yet, serious AD in fattening pigs has
rarely been attributed to the introduction of weaners from
infected breeding herds. This is probably because the virus is
similar to the NIA 1 strain which is relatively non virulent
in fattening pigs (Baskerville et al., 1973).

     AD in these herds often appears to be related in some
way to the pigs suffering some stress, such as changes in the
quality of feed or fluctuating temperature. Therefore control
of AD in these situations is brought about by a combination of
vaccine and the elimination of the stress factor.

     Only nine fattening herds have used vaccine. This small
number reflects the relative unimportance of the disease in
fattening herds. In the majority of these herds it has not
been necessary to follow a continuous programme of vaccination.
Instead, vaccine is usually used following the appearance of
AD among the fattening pigs and it may be discontinued after a
period of time. In other fattening herds the manufacturers'
directions for the use of vaccine have not even been followed

and only one of the two recommended injections of vaccine has been administered.

Over the last 15 months since AD vaccine was first introduced there have been only a few reported cases of AD in breeding herds. These have involved weaner pigs of six weeks and older. Morbidity and mortality have been low. Serological investigations in these herds have demonstrated variable titres in the sow population and thus disease in these weaners can be associated with waning maternal immunity.

As vaccine has only been in use for a relatively short period of time, its role in AD control awaits further evaluation. However, careful monitoring of the disease over the next decade should allow a more critical appraisal of its value.

REFERENCE

Baskerville, A., McFerran, J.B. and Dow, C., 1973. Aujeszky's disease in pigs. Vet. Bull. 43, 465-480.

COMPARATIVE STUDIES WITH INACTIVATED AND ATTENUATED VACCINES FOR PROTECTION OF FATTENING PIGS

J.B. McFerran, R.M. McCracken and C. Dow

Veterinary Research Laboratories, Stormont,
Belfast BT4 3SD, Northern Ireland.

ABSTRACT

Six inactivated and three attenuated vaccines were compared. Pigs were inoculated with vaccine and after 2 weeks challenged by intranasal inoculation of NIA 3 virus. Excellent protection was given by the attenuated and some of the inactivated vaccines tested. None prevented the challenge virus being excreted, but they did reduce the amount shed.

INTRODUCTION

Although antibody to Aujeszky's disease virus (ADV) is relatively widespread amongst pigs in Northern Ireland, it is generally not a major disease problem. Typically sporadic outbreaks are seen, causing deaths in young pigs and abortions and stillbirths in pregnant animals. However, once the clinical disease has subsided within 2 - 4 weeks, the disease may not reappear for many years. There are between 10 and 30 outbreaks a year diagnosed at the Veterinary Laboratories.

In 1972, however, a severe outbreak was seen in a large fattening unit, where mortality in 12 - 16 week old pigs due to ADV reached 13%. This outbreak was controlled by the use of a Bartha strain vaccine prepared at Stormont (McFerran and Dow, 1975) and subsequent breakdowns in this herd have been controlled by an attenuated NIA 4 vaccine also made at Stormont. Recently there have been a number of outbreaks in other fattening units, leading to a policy decision that whilst eradication should be encouraged in pedigree breeding units, vaccination was desirable to control disease in commercial units.

Whilst some fattening units obtain their pigs from recognised sources, allowing a vaccination programme to be established, most buy their pigs on the open market. As the disease tends to occur between 2 and 4 weeks after the introduction of pigs onto the farm, clearly one dose of vaccine will have to produce good immunity within 2 weeks.

G. Wittmann, S.A. Hall (eds), Aujeszky's Disease. ISBN-13:978-94-009-7555-2

Therefore an experiment was carried out to compare two attenuated vaccines (the BUK and NIA 4) and an oil adjuvant vaccine (McFerran et al., 1979). All three vaccines gave a good immunity. The present communication reports the continuation of this work to evaluate a number of commercial or experimental vaccines for use in protecting fattening pigs.

MATERIALS AND METHODS

Pigs

These were obtained from a herd of pigs established by caesarian section and free of antibody to or clinical signs of Aujeszky's disease (AD). Following weaning at 3 weeks of age, they were moved to the experimental accommodation and randomly distributed into groups for vaccination at 5 - 6 weeks of age.

Challenge virus

One ml of the NIA 3 strain of virulent ADV was given intranasally. Each pig received 10^6 tissue culture infective doses fifty ($TCID_{50}$) of virus. The pigs were challenged 2 weeks following vaccination. Control pigs from the same litters and kept in the same house as the vaccinates were also infected.

Determination of virus neutralising antibody and virus isolation

The methods used were as described (McFerran et al., 1979). Blood samples were taken before vaccination (0 weeks), before challenge (2 weeks) and 3 weeks after challenge.

Vaccines

The following vaccines were used. The volume and route of vaccine administered was that suggested by the manufacturer. The number of pigs used is given in Table 1.

Experiment 1

Four vaccines were compared. Two were commercially available inactivated vaccines, one from Laboratoire Roger Bellon,

TABLE 1

MORTALITY FOLLOWING INTRANASAL CHALLENGE OF PIGS WITH VIRULENT AUJESZKY'S DISEASE VIRUS

Treatment	Number of pigs		Per cent mortality	Number dying on day					
	Vaccinated	Died		4	5	6	7	9	10
Experiment 1									
Vaccine A	14	O	O			O			
Vaccine B	15	13	87	3	8	-	2		
Vaccine C	15	3	23	1	-	1	-	1	-
Vaccine NIA 4	15	O	O			O			
Control	14	12	86	6	4	2	-	-	-
Experiment 2									
Vaccine D	16	2	12.5	-	-	-	1	1	-
Vaccine E	16	O	O			O			
Vaccine F	16	1	6.25	-	-	1	-	-	-
Vaccine Bartha	16	O	O			O			
Vaccine NIA 4	15	O	O			O			
Control	22	21	95	-	2	12	5	1	1

France, and the other from Salsbury Laboratories, USA; the third was an experimental inactivated vaccine from Intervet, The Netherlands, and the fourth was an experimental attenuated NIA 4 vaccine. The NIA 4 vaccine contained $10^{6.5}$ TCID$_{50}$/ml.

Experiment 2

Five vaccines were tested. Two were commercially available vaccines, one from Norden Laboratories, USA, and the other from Intervet Laboratories, The Netherlands. The others were an experimental inactivated vaccine from Duphar, The Netherlands; a commercially available attenuated vaccine, Bartha strain also from Duphar, and an experimental attenuated NIA 4 vaccine. The NIA 4 vaccine in this trial contained $10^{5.5}$ TCID$_{50}$/ml.

RESULTS

The vaccinated pigs remained healthy during the 2 week observation period. Following challenge the control pigs

developed typical signs of AD. Body temperature became elevated
on the 2nd or 3rd days (Table 2). The pigs were dull, dis-
inclined to move and had a greatly reduced food intake. These
symptoms intensified over 24 h and many pigs became depressed.
Some pigs vomited and most had the typical hoarse squeal when
handled. Nervous signs, initially shown by muscle twitching,
became more pronounced with incoordination or ataxia, and
behavioural changes such as aimlessly walking in circles or
biting at boots or straw. Pigs developed lateral recumbency,
frequently paddling with all 4 legs or having convulsions.
Peak mortality was seen between days 4 and 7 (Table 1).

TABLE 2

MEAN TEMPERATURES FOLLOWING CHALLENGES WITH VIRULENT AUJESZKY'S DISEASE VIRUS

	Mean body temperature				Days post challenge		
	2	3	4	5	6	7	8
Experiment 1							
A	-	105.9	105.9	104.2	104	102.5	102.3
B	-	105.2	105.1	105.1	104.2	103.5	101.8
C	-	106.4	106.9	105.5	105.6	104.5	103.5
NIA 4	-	104.9	105.3	103.6	103.1	102.6	102.5
Control	-	105.3	105.8	106.2	104	100.8	101.4
Experiment 2							
D	104.0	106	106.1	105.9	104.9	103.4	103.4
E	105.3	105.6	105.6	105.5	103.8	103.1	102.5
F	104.3	104.7	105.1	106.1	106	103.6	103.5
Bartha	103.9	104.2	104.3	103.3	102.2	102.8	102.6
NIA 4	105.5	105.8	105.6	104.3	102.2	102.6	102.3
Control	105.5	105.6	105.2	104.7	101.2	-	-

In the first experiment the pigs inoculated with vaccine
B were clinically indistinguishable from the controls and their
mortality rates were similar (Table 1). The pigs vaccinated
with A or C developed elevated temperatures on the 3rd day after
challenge (Table 2). They were constipated, showed a reduced
food intake and were reluctant to move. Some pigs showed

transient nervous signs. Although 3 of the pigs vaccinated with C died and the group as a whole had higher mean body temperatures than group A the pigs in group C appeared less severely affected. Apart from a mild temperature rise and some reluctance to eat their full ration on days 3 and 4 p.c., the NIA 4 group were unaffected.

In the second experiment pigs vaccinated with D were quite ill. The whole group was not eating on 4th day post challenge and most did not eat on 5th d.p.c. They had the highest temperatures of any group (Table 2). They were very depressed and even by 8th d.p.c. were not active and 3 pigs were still rubbing their noses on the floor. Two pigs died, one on day 7 and the other on day 9. The pigs infected with vaccine E were much brighter. They had a transient inappetence on 4th d.p.c. and showed some depression and voice change. Vaccine group F became dull on 2nd d.p.c. and rejected their food on the 4th d.p.c. On day 5, most had marked voice changes and one pig showed definite signs of pruritus. The NIA 4 group this time were quite ill. All refused their food on the 3rd and 4th d.p.c. and nervous signs were seen in two pigs. In contrast the group vaccinated with the Bartha strain were clinically the healthiest pigs with only some voice change on 4th d.p.c.

All groups of pigs excreted virus when challenged with virulent virus (Table 3). All the pigs given inactivated vaccines excreted virus fairly constantly for the first 8 days with between 60 and 80% of the swabs positive.

An exception was the pigs given vaccine D, where only 42% were positive and those given B where there was no reduction in virus excretion compared to the controls. The groups given attenuated vaccine showed a marked reduction in the excretion of the challenge virus. This was especially true of the Bartha infected pigs, where only 27% of swabs were positive.

None of the pigs used in these experiments had any detectable antibody before vaccination. After vaccination the geometric mean titres varied from 1.2 to 13.9 (Table 4). With most vaccines tested detectable antibody did not develop in every pig within the 2 week period before challenge. Exceptions

were the pigs given vaccines C, F and the higher titre NIA 4
vaccine, where every pig had titres of at least 1/2.

TABLE 3

DETECTION OF VIRUS IN THE NASAL EXCRETIONS OF PIGS INFECTED WITH VIRULENT
VIRUS, IN THE FIRST 8 DAYS POST CHALLENGE

Treatment	Number of samples			% positive
	Tested	Positive	Negative	
Experiment 1				
Vaccine A	40	28	12	70
Vaccine B	27*	24	3	88.9
Vaccine C	40	34	6	85
Vaccine NIA 4	40	20	20	50
Control	25*	24	1	96
Experiment 2				
Vaccine D	64	29	35	42.2
Vaccine E	64	40	24	62.5
Vaccine F	60*	38	22	63.3
Vaccine Bartha	64	17	47	26.6
Vaccine NIA 4	64	31	33	48.4
Control	75*	63	12	84

* Fewer samples taken because of mortality in these groups.

DISCUSSION

With the exception of vaccine B, all these vaccines
induced good to excellent protection against ADV. This was
rather surprising as only one injection was given and only 2
weeks were allowed for immunity to develop before challenge.
All the vaccine manufacturers recommended two doses of vaccine
usually given 4 weeks apart. This programme may be ideal, but
is impractical with the disease problem and husbandry problems
encountered in the fied.

The pigs vaccinated with Bartha vaccine excreted less
virus than any other group. They were also the most healthy
group after challenge, showing only some voice change on one
day after challenge and they had the lowest rise in body

TABLE 4

RESULTS OF TESTING SERA FOR NEUTRALISING ANTIBODY FROM VACCINATED PIGS
BEFORE AND AFTER CHALLENGE WITH VIRULENT AUJESZKY'S DISEASE VIRUS

| Vaccine | SN titre | | | |
| | Pre challenge | | Post challenge | |
	Mean	Range	Mean	Range
Experiment 1				
A	6.6	2–32	156	128–256
B	1.3	2–4	209	128–256
C	12.7	4–32	228	128–512
NIA 4	13.9	4–32	370	256–1024
Experiment 2				
D	1.2	2–6	153	96–256
E	2.3	2–12	231	128–512
F	9.0	4–32	387	256–512
Bartha	4.8	2–12	293	128–512
NIA 4	1.4	2–24	146	16–768

* Titres are expressed as the reciprocal of the final serum dilution which
neutralises 100 $TCID_{50}$ (30 – 300) of virus.

NB No antibody was detected in the pre-vaccination sera.

temperature. The group vaccinated with $10^{6.5}$ NIA 4 vaccine also
remained clinically healthy apart from some degree of inappetence
and a temperature rise. The group given 10 times less virus,
however, were ill, although no worse than most groups given
inactivated vaccine and all the pigs survived. There appears
to be a correlation between the vaccine virus titre and immunity.
A similar correlation has been noted by others (Jamrichova and
Skoda, 1969).

No vaccine was able to prevent the challenge virus from
growing in the nasal mucosa, so therefore all these pigs could
become potential carriers. However most vaccines reduced the
amount of virulent virus being excreted. This was especially
true of the attenuated Bartha virus strain.

The serum antibody titres found 2 weeks after vaccination
gave little guide to the potency of the vaccine. Thus whilst

vaccines D, E and NIA 4 (low dose) gave good protection with low geometric mean titres (GMT), vaccine B with a similar GMT gave no discernible protection. Furthermore using vaccine C, with one of the highest GMTs, there was a 23% mortality. Vaccine D had the lowest GMT, and although there was a 12.5% mortality, these pigs excreted less challenge virus than any other group vaccinated with inactivated vaccine.

This represents a problem in licensing inactivated vaccines. If the antibody response is not a useful parameter what can be used to measure the potency of the vaccine? In the case of attenuated vaccines, the virus titre appears to be a good and easily established guide to its potency.

On many grounds attenuated vaccines, if suitable strains are selected, would appear to be the vaccine of choice for immunising fattening pigs. Thus the BUK (Jamrichova and Skoda, 1969), the Bartha (Bartha and Kojnok, 1963; McFerran and Dow, 1975) and the NIA 4 strain (McFerran and Dow, unpublished; Zygraich, 1978) are not excreted. If grown in semi-continuous cell lines and if the source of serum is controlled and if versene is used in place of trypsin, then the risk of contamination can be greatly reduced. Furthermore it is relatively easy to test attenuated vaccines, whilst inactivated vaccines with adjuvant are very difficult to test in cell culture systems.

Further work is in progress on the use of these vaccines in the presence of maternal antibody. Preliminary work suggests that the attenuated vaccines may well be capable of stimulating adequate immunity.

REFERENCES

Bartha, A. and Kojnok, J., 1963. Active immunisation against Aujeszky's disease. Proc. 17th Wld. Vet. Cong. Hanover 1, 531-533.
Jamrichova, O. and Skoda, R., 1969. Multiplication and distribution of attenuated pseudorabies virus in the organisms of vaccinated pigs. Acta Virologica. 13, 42-51
McFerran, J.B. and Dow, C., 1975. Studies on immunisation of pigs with the Bartha strain of Aujeszky's disease virus. Res. Vet Sci., 19, 17-22.
McFerran, J.B., Dow, C. and McCracken, R.M., 1979. Experimental studies in weaned pigs with three vaccines against Aujeszky's Disease. Comp. Immun. Microbio. Infect. Dis., 2, 327-334.
Zygraich, N., 1978. Rit. Genval Belgium, personal communication.

EARLY PROTECTION AFTER VACCINATION AGAINST AUJESZKY'S DISEASE

J.T. van Oirschot, P.W. de Leeuw and D. van Zaane

Central Veterinary Institute, Department of Virology,
39, Houtribweg, 8221 RA Lelystad, The Netherlands.

ABSTRACT

To determine how soon protection against Aujeszky's disease (AD) is induced, pigs were vaccinated with a modified live virus vaccine or an inactivated vaccine, and challenged intranasally with a virulent strain of Aujeszky's disease virus (ADV) after 2, 4 or 6 days. After 2 - 4 days the vaccinated pigs were already partially protected, as shown by a lower mortality, a less severe course of disease and a reduced excretion of virulent virus as compared to that in the control pigs. Both vaccines appeared to be equally effective in producing an early protection.

Sensitised peripheral blood lymphocytes and/or low levels of neutralising antibody, were detected in some pigs on day 6 after vaccination. No interferon was found in the sera of any of the vaccinated pigs. Possible mechanisms underlying the early protective immunity are discussed.

INTRODUCTION

Vaccination during an outbreak of Aujeszky's disease (AD) in pig herds can reduce the appearance of new cases within 5 - 10 days (Bartha and Kojnok, 1963; Zuffa and Polak, 1965). These observations suggest an early protective effect of vaccination against AD. Under experimental conditions, vaccine potency is usually examined at least 2 weeks after vaccination. Only a few experimental data are available on the early immunity induced by Aujeszky's disease virus (ADV) vaccines (Wittmann and Jakubik, 1977; Tatarov, 1978).

The objective of this study was to determine the degree of protection in pigs when challenged 2, 4 or 6 days after vaccination with a modified live virus (MLV) vaccine or an inactivated vaccine.

MATERIALS AND METHODS

Pigs

Pigs were from the Dutch Landrace minimal disease herd of the Central Veterinary Institute. The herd is free of antibodies to ADV. In each of two similar experiments 20 10-week-old pigs were randomly divided into 4 groups of 5. Three groups were vaccinated 6, 4 or 2 days before challenge. One group remained unvaccinated and served as a control. Pigs were observed daily for clinical signs; rectal temperatures were also recorded daily. The pigs were weighed 1 week before challenge and thereafter three times a week.

Vaccination and challenge exposure

In the first experiment vaccination was done with a MLV vaccine (MK-25, Pharmachim, Bulgaria); in the second experiment an inactivated oil adjuvant vaccine (Nobivac, Intervet International B.V., Boxmeer, The Netherlands) was used. Vaccinations were performed according to the manufacturers' instructions. The Northern Ireland Three (NIA-3) strain (McFerran and Dow, 1975) kindly provided by Dr. J.B. McFerran, Stormont, Belfast, Northern Ireland, was used as challenge virus. This strain was passaged six times in secondary pig kidney (PK_2) cells. The pigs were challenged by administering 0.5 ml of the virus suspension (containing 10^5 plaque forming units (p.f.u.)/ml) into each nostril. The pigs were given a tranquilliser (Stresnil, Janssen Pharmaceutica, Beerse, Belgium) before challenge.

Collection and processing of samples

Blood samples were drawn from the anterior *vena cava* on days 6, 4, 3 and 2 before challenge, on the day of challenge and, in the groups given the inactivated vaccine, on days 3, 7, 14 and 21 after challenge. For lymphocyte stimulation studies, blood was drawn into tubes containing preservative-free heparin. Oropharyngeal (OP) fluids were collected as described previously (De Leeuw et al., 1979) but 4 ml of buffer was added to the swabs and arctone extraction was omitted. OP swabs were taken daily after vaccination with the MLV vaccine and for 10 consecutive days after challenge.

Virus titration and virus neutralisation test

OP samples were assayed for virus as described (De leeuw et al., 1979). Sera were tested for neutralising antibody in

duplicate in a microtitre system, using PK_2 cells and a serum/
virus incubation period of 24 h at $37^{\circ}C$ (Bitsch and Eskildsen,
1976). Serum titres are expressed as the log_{10} of the reciprocal
of the highest dilution inhibiting cytopathic effect in 50% of
the cultures.

Lymphocyte stimulation

The mitogenic and antigenic lymphocyte stimulation tests
with peripheral blood mononuclear cells were performed as
described previously (Van Oirschot, 1978). In the mitogenic
lymphocyte stimulation test a concentration of 0.5% phytohaem-
agglutinin (PHA) (HA15, Wellcome, Beckenham, England) was used.
In the antigenic lymphocyte stimulation test 1 ml of antigen
was equivalent to 7.5 p.f.u. of ADV. The mean stimulation index
(SI) + 2.SD calculated from 100 determinations in seronegative
pigs was 3.22, (mean SI ± SD: 1.18 ± 1.02). Therefore we considered a SI ≥ 3.3 to be positive.

Test for interferon

Sera, taken 2, 4 or 6 days after vaccination, were tested
for the presence of interferon, according to standard methods,
using a plaque reduction test on PK_2 cells with vesicular
stomatitis virus as indicator virus.

RESULTS

No clinical signs or elevated temperatures were noticed
after vaccination with either the MLV or the inactivated vaccine.
After challenge, control as well as vaccinated pigs developed
signs of illness, but those in vaccinated pigs were less severe
and of shorter duration. The most pronounced symptoms were
high fever, dullness, loss of appetite, vomiting, sneezing,
nasal discharge, difficult respiration and nervous symptoms
such as lack of co-ordination and epileptiform convulsions. In
both experiments 3 out of 5 control pigs died on days 6 or 7
after challenge, whereas the mortality in the vaccinated groups
was markedly lower or absent (Table 1).

TABLE 1

PROTECTION OF VACCINATED PIGS AGAINST CHALLENGE WITH VIRULENT ADV.

Vaccine	Days between vaccination and challenge	Number[1] that died	Days of[2] fever	Days of[3] arrested growth
Modified live	6	0	2	3
	4	1	6	6
	2	1	4	5.5
	controls	3	6	7
Inactivated	6	0	5	8
	4	0	6	9
	2	1	7	12
	controls	3	6	15

[1] Each group consisted of 5 10-week-old pigs
[2] Mean body temperature of the group $\geq 40^{\circ}C$
[3] Number of days survivors needed to regain the mean weight on day 1 after challenge

The duration of fever and the mean body temperatures were approximately the same in the different groups, with the exception of pigs vaccinated with the MLV vaccine 6 days before challenge (Table 1).

The develoment of body weight is an objective parameter to evaluate protection against a virulent infection with ADV. The mean weight curves of the pigs involved in the second experiment are depicted in Figure 1. This figure shows that the control pigs had their maximum loss of weight on day 8 post challenge. The period of growth arrest (the period needed to regain the starting weight on day 1 post challenge) was shorter in the vaccinated pigs than in the controls. In addition, shorter periods of growth arrest were found when pigs had been vaccinated earlier before challenge.

In groups of pigs given the MLV vaccine, basically the same pattern was found (data not shown).

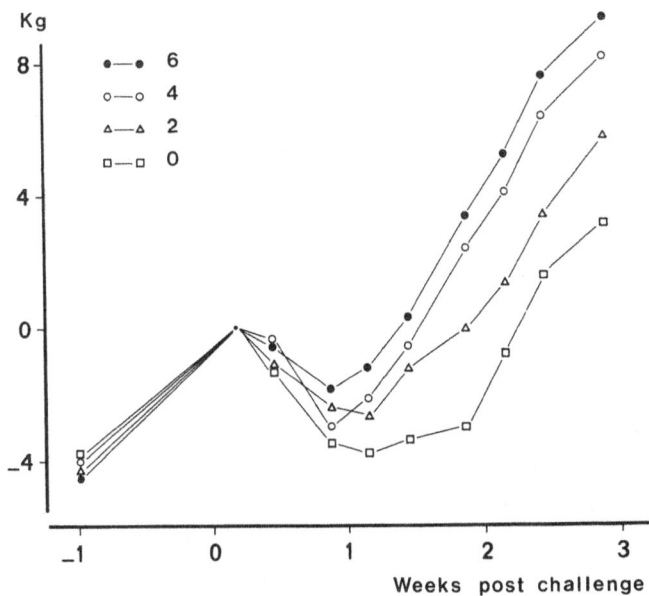

Fig. 1. Mean weight curves of groups of 5 pigs vaccinated with the
inactivated vaccine 6, 4 or 2 days before challenge. One
group served as control (O).

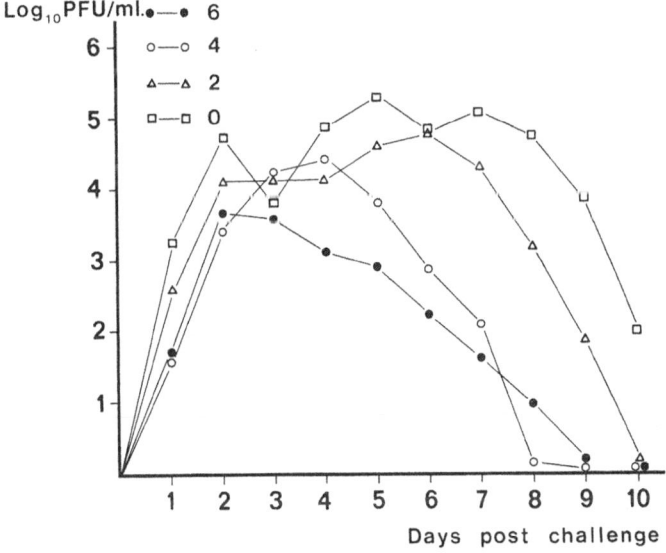

Fig. 2. Mean virus titres in oro-pharyngeal fluids of groups of
4 pigs given the inactivated vaccine 6, 4 or 2 days before
challenge. One group was not vaccinated (O).

Figure 2 shows the mean virus titres per ml of OP fluid of pigs vaccinated with the vaccine during 10 days after challenge. Particularly after the third day post challenge, the quantity of virus in OP secretions was considerably reduced as compared to that in controls, the reduction being greatest in pigs given the vaccine 6 days before challenge. Moreover, vaccinated pigs excreted virus for shorter periods than control pigs.

Pigs vaccinated with the MLV vaccine also excreted less virus in OP fluids than controls. No virus was recovered from OP fluids of these pigs in the period between vaccination and challenge.

On day 6 post vaccination, low levels of neutralising anti-body were found in the sera of 2 out of the 5 pigs that had received the inactivated vaccine. On days 2 and 4 post vaccin-ation all pigs were negative. Moderate titres were detected on day 3 and high titres on day 7 after challenge in the pigs vaccinated 6 or 4 days before challenge. Titres increased markedly more slowly in control pigs (Figure 3).

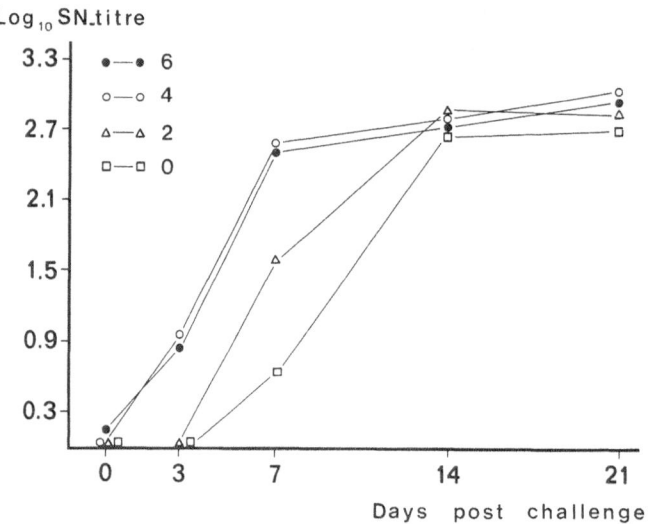

Fig. 3. Mean serum neutralising antibody titres in groups of
        5 pigs given the inactivated vaccine 6, 4 or 2 days
        before challenge. One groups was not vaccinated (0).

Of all pigs vaccinated with the MLV vaccine, only 1 had neutralising antibody on day 6 post vaccination.

addition, vaccinated pigs had lower virus titres in OP fluids
and excreted virulent virus for shorter periods than controls.
Judging from the number of pigs that died after challenge, both
vaccines appeared equally effective. The growth arrest periods
of the groups vaccinated with the MLV vaccine were shorter than
those of the 'comparable' groups vaccinated with the inactivated
vaccine, but the same held true for the controls. Therefore,
the results do not allow a conclusion as to which vaccine was
most effective in inducing an early protection.

The above results, in general, confirm and extend those of
others. Wittmann and Jakubik (1977) reported almost complete
protection in pigs challenged 7 days after the administration of
an experimental inactivated vaccine with diethylaminoethyl-
dextrane (DEAE-D) as adjuvant. They had not tested the degree
of protection earlier after vaccination. Tatarov (1978) found
that the same MLV vaccine as used in this study, prevented death
in pigs challenged beyond 4 days after vaccination.

The immune mechanisms underlying the early protection
observed after vaccination against AD are not clear. A role for
interferon is unlikely, because no interferon activity was
demonstrated. In addition, virulent ADV appeared to have little
sensitivity to interferon (Wawrzkiewicz, 1966; Lomniczi, 1974).
Humoral immunity, as such, does not appear to be a major factor
in the protective mechanism, because low levels of neutralising
antibody were detected in only 3 pigs on the day of challenge.
Nevertheless, pigs vaccinated 4 - 6 days before challenge were
sensitised as indicated by a secondary type neutralising antibody response. This implies the presence of antigen-responsive
lymphocytes in these pigs. With the lymphocyte stimulation test
we found antigen-reactive lymphocytes in the blood from only 3
pigs, on the day of challenge. However, most antigen-reactive
lymphocytes are probably located in the lymphnodes draining the
injected area. Based on the above, it appears that at least one
of the mechanisms involved in the observed early protection
against AD is the development of sensitised lymphocytes. These
sensitised lymphocytes react rapidly upon re-exposure to ADV
antigens and the resulting secondary type of immune response,
then quickly inhibit virus multiplication before widespread

damage of tissues ensues.

Our experimental findings substantiate observations in the field that vaccination shortly after the onset of an outbreak of AD can reduce the severity of clinical signs and can prevent the appearance of new cases. Theoretical drawbacks of such an interfering vaccination could be activation of sub-clinical ADV infections, and of ADV infections in the incubation period. However, it has been shown that an inactivated vaccine with DEAE-D adjuvant given during the incubation period of an ADV infection did not influence the frequency and severity of clinical signs (Jakubik and Wittmann, 1978).

ACKNOWLEDGEMENTS

We thank D. de Jong, W.A.M. van Rossum and J.W.A. Tiessink for skilful technical assistance.

REFERENCES

Bartha, A. and Kojnok, J. 1963. Active immunization against Aujeszky's disease. Proc. 17th Wld vet. Congr., Hannover 1, 531-533.

Bitsch, V. and Eskildsen, M. 1976. A comparative examination of swine sera for antibody to Aujeszky virus with the conventional and a modified virus-serum neutralization test and a modified direct complement fixation test. Acta Vet. Scand., 17, 142-152.

De Leeuw, P.W., Tiessink, J.W.A. and Van Bekkum, J.G. 1979. The challenge of vaccinated pigs with foot-and-mouth disease virus. Zbl. Vet. Med. B, 26, 98-108.

Jakubik, J. and Wittmann, G. 1978. Schutzimpfung mit inaktivierter Aujeszky-virus (AV)-Vakzine in der Inkubationszeit einer AV-Infektion. Versuch, eine Provokation der Infektion auszulösen. Dtsch. Tierärtzl. Wschr., 85, 285-288.

Lomniczi, B. 1974. Biological properties of Aujeszky's disease (Pseudo-rabies) virus strains with special regard to interferon production and interferon sensitivity. Arch. ges. Virusforschung, 44, 205-214.

McFerran, J.B. and Dow, C. 1975. Studies on immunisation of pigs with the Bartha strain of Aujeszky's disease virus. Res. Vet. Sci., 19, 17-22.

Tatarov, G. 1978. The virus of Aujeszky's disease. Zemizdat, Sofia, Bulgaria.

Van Oirschot, J.T. 1978. In vitro stimulation of pig lymphocytes after infection and vaccination with Aujeszky's disease virus. Vet. Microbiol., 3, 255-268.

Wawrzkiewicz, J. 1966. Interferon formation by strains of Aujeskzy's disease virus. Medycyna wet., 22, 657-660.

Wittmann, G. and Jakubik, J. 1977. Frühstadium der Immunität nach Impfung von Ferkeln mit einer inaktivierten Aujeszkyvirus-Vakzine. Zbl. Vet. Med. B., 569-575.

Zuffa, A. and Polak, V. 1965. Immunoprophylaxie de certaines maladies à virus du porc et des volailles en Tchécoslovaquie. Bull. Off. int. Epizoot. 64, 297-307.

EFFICIENCY OF AN INACTIVATED VIRUS VACCINE AGAINST AUJESZKY'S DISEASE FOR FATTENING PIGS WITH OR WITHOUT PASSIVE IMMUNITY

P. Vannier

Ministère de l'Agriculture, Direction de la Qualité,
Services Vétérinaires, Station de Pathologie Porcine,
BP n° 9 22440 Ploufragan, France.

ABSTRACT

   In an attempt to understand the real causes of respiratory problems in fattening units of the breeding and fattening herds infected by Aujeszky's disease virus (ADV) and the reasons of the apparent inefficiency of the inactivated virus vaccine used in France in these cases, an experimental study was done. Three groups of 5 month old fattening pigs were challenged with a virulent ADV strain. In one group, pigs were not vaccinated and were born from non-vaccinated sows; in another one, pigs were vaccinated and were born from vaccinated sows; in the last one, pigs were vaccinated against Aujeszky's disease (AD) but were born from non-vaccinated sows. The results of the experiment showed that this vaccine gives a relative protection to fattening pigs against this particular form of AD, but only in the absence of passive immunity. A marked difference appeared between the three groups if the clinical signs, the weight losses and the time necessary for recovering the initial weight are considered. The presence of maternal antibodies and the level of passive immunity are the main factors which determine the development of an active immunity after vaccination. However, it seems that the sanitary status of pigs before infection with ADV has an effect on the intensity of clinical reactions of the infected animals. ADV causes a severe depression of the pigs' condition which favours the onset of a bacterial infection. Conditions leading to the onset of this particular form of AD in fattening units are examined and measures for avoiding the onset of these problems are discussed.

INTRODUCTION

   It is a fact that Aujeszky's disease (AD) is causing more and more problems and economic losses in fattening units on breeding and fattening farms. The situation is confused in the field and it is difficult to appreciate exactly the evolution of the disease and the cause of the troubles in the fattening units. The inactivated virus vaccine used in France* seems to be inefficient for protecting the fattening pigs against this particular form of AD. In an attempt to clarify this situation, an experimental study was made by reproducing the natural conditions of the onset of AD in fattening units.

* Geskyvac Laboratoire Roger Bellon

G. Wittmann, S.A. Hall (eds), Aujeszky's Disease. ISBN-13:978-94-009-7555-2

To this end, three groups of 5 month old fattening pigs were challenged with a virulent ADV strain. In the first group, the pigs were not vaccinated against AD and were born from non-vaccinated sows; in the second group, the pigs were vaccinated and born from vaccinated sows; in the third group, the pigs were vaccinated against AD but were born from non-vaccinated sows.

MATERIALS AND METHODS

Animals

The pigs were divided into three groups as shown in Table 1.

TABLE 1

DESCRIPTION OF THE EXPERIMENT

Group		Number of pigs	Pigs born from sow no.	Age at vaccination	Age at challenge
non	A	6	1 and 2	no vaccination	22 weeks
vaccinated	a	7 (Ba)	1 and 2	10 weeks	22 weeks
sows 1 - 2	B				
	b	6 (Bb)	1 and 2	17 weeks	22 weeks
vaccinated	a	10 (Ca)	3 and 4	11 weeks	23 weeks
sows 3 - 4	C				
	b	10 (Cb)	3 and 4	18 weeks	23 weeks

Sows 1 and 2 were bought from a conventional herd in which neither the breeders nor the baconers were vaccinated against AD. No AD neutralising antibody was found either in the serum of these sows or of the other sows of the herd.

Sows 3 and 4 had been bought from a conventional herd in which the breeders were regularly vaccinated (Geskyvac) against AD. The baconers were not vaccinated and serological investigations in the fattening units did not reveal the presence of neutralising antibodies. No clinical sign of AD was ever observed in the herd.

Sows 3 and 4 had already farrowed more than 5 litters and had been vaccinated before each weaning.

The 4 sows were pregnant on arrival at the research centre and each group of sows was housed in isolation from the others. Airtight panels separated each section; the air was filtered through absolute filters. Each sow farrowed in isolation. After weaning the piglets were randomised; the pigs of each group (A, Ba, Bb, Ca, Cb) were housed in pens isolated from the others. In each, the housing conditions were optimal (constant temperature, low air speed, high air volume).

Fattening pigs' vaccination

The 13 pigs born from the non vaccinated sows 1 - 2 were vaccinated when they were 10 weeks old (Ba) and 17 weeks old (Bb). The other 20 pigs born from sows 3 - 4 vaccinated against AD, were vaccinated when they were 11 weeks old (Ca) and 18 weeks old (Cb). Each pig was given 2 ml of the vaccine by the intramuscular route.

Challenge

All the pigs from the three groups were challenged when they were 22 to 23 weeks old.

In the present study, challenge was performed nasally with the 75 v 19 strain from Belgium (Andries et al., 1978). Each pig, received 4 ml of the virulent ADV containing $10^{6.7}$ $TCID_{50}$/ml.

Pathological examinations

Each pig that died naturally or was killed, was examined for gross lesions. Samples of lungs and tonsils were collected on killed pigs for virological investigations.

Serological studies

Inactivated sera (30 minutes at 56°C) were examined for seroneutralising antibodies by preparing two-fold dilutions in a Microtitre plate.

The dilutions were mixed with an equal volume of ADV containing approximately 100 $TCID_{50}$. After 1 hour of

incubation at 37°C, approximately 24 000 cells of the PK 15
cell line were seeded in each well. The reciprocal of the
highest dilution of the serum which completely neutralised
the virus, as indicated by the absence of cytopathic effect,
was considered as the titre. The final titre was determined
after 5 days and was expressed in the initial dilution of the
serum.

Clinical observations

The clinical signs, especially the respiratory disorders,
and the rectal temperatures were recorded daily. Each pig was
weighed once a week; the weight loss and the length of the
pyrexia were the main criteria used for evaluation of the
protection.

RESULTS

Clinical observations. Pathological examinations

Group A (Control)

Two days after challenge, all the pigs showed marked
and persistent hyperthermia (> 41°C, more than 9 days). They
became prostrate and showed respiratory disorders (dyspnoea,
cough, sneezing). Before challenge, no clinical signs had
been observed.

Seven days after challenge, 2 pigs died. A third one
died, but not until 21 days after the first ones. The 2 pigs
which died soon after challenge showed congestion of the tonsils and lymphnodes with a very slight pleuritis. The third
one presented much more marked lesions than the others: congestion of the tonsils, purulent pneumonia and extensive pleuritis.
On the 3 survivors, killed 40 days after challenge, different
lesions were observed: purulent pneumonia, pleuritis, congestion
of the lymphnodes.

Group B (born from non-vaccinated sows)

After challenge, the pigs in group Ba (vaccinated when

10 weeks old) showed a marked hyperthermia (>40.5°C) but it
lasted no longer than 3 days and the pigs were prostrate for
only 3 days. No other clinical sign was observed in these 7
pigs and no lesion was observed at necropsy when they were
killed 57 days after inoculation.

The pigs in group Bb (vaccinated when 17 weeks old) showed more intense clinical signs than those in group Ba: the
hyperthermia lasted 3 days but the respiratory disorders were
marked and lasted 10 days at least. These clinical signs were
not apparent before challenge. One pig died 7 days after inoculation with different lesions: congestion of the tonsils,
lymphnodes, peritonitis, ascitis.

No lesion was observed in the survivors killed 57 days
after inoculation.

Group C (born from vaccinated sows)

After challenge the pigs in group Ca (vaccinated at 11
weeks old) showed a really marked hyperthermia ($\geqslant 41$°C) which
lasted 9 days in all the pigs. They became prostrate, showed
dyspnoea and anorexia. Respiratory disorders were slight. In
fact, one pig died 3 days after challenge with a massive nasal
haemorrhage.

When the 9 survivors were killed, 30 days after inoculation, different lesions were observed; among 6 of them, pneumonia pleuritis and pericarditis were observed. The other 3
showed no lesion at necropsy.

In group Cb (vaccinated at 18 weeks old) the hyperthermia
following challenge lasted only 4 days on the 6 pigs born from
sow 3 whereas it lasted more than 8 days on the 4 pigs born
from sow 4. A marked dyspnoea was observed on pig 1 and frequent sneezing was heard. The prostrated state of the pigs
lasted as long as the hyperthermia persisted.

At necropsy, pleuritis was observed in 5 pigs. No
lesion was observed in the others.

Weight losses (Table 2)

The weight losses were very high in the control group.
A marked difference was observed between the control group
and groups B and C. Nevertheless, a difference in reaction
was clearly observed between groups B and C. The weight
losses were lower in group B than in group C; moreover, the
period of time necessary for recovering the initial weight is an
important factor. This period of time is shorter in group B
than in group C which shows clearly a relative efficiency of
the vaccine when used without passive immunity.

TABLE 2

PERFORMANCES OF THE DIFFERENT GROUPS AFTER CHALLENGE

Group	Mean daily growth BC	Total weight losses AC by pig	Mean daily growth 6 days AC	Mean daily growth 21 days AC	Time necessary for recovering the initial weight
A (control)	864 g	17.8 kg	(− 1800 g)	(− 572 g)	no recovery > 36 days
B* (vaccina- a ted at 10 weeks	864 g	5 kg	(− 833 g)	+ 300 g	10 days
(vaccina- b ted at 17 weeks)	890 g	4.5 kg	(− 750 g)	+ 476 g	10 days
C** (vaccina- a ted at 11 weeks)	704 g	7 kg	(− 1166 g)	− 75 g	20 days
(vaccina- b ted at 18 weeks)	803 g	7 kg	(− 1166 g)	200 g	17 days

* (non-vaccinated sows)   AC: After Challenge

** (vaccinated sow)   BC: Before Challenge

Serological investigations

Tables 3 and 4 show the mean titre of the antibodies in
the sera of the animals in groups A and B.

TABLE 3

SEROLOGICAL STUDIES IN GROUPS A AND B (MEAN TITRE IN EACH GROUP)

										Age of pigs (weeks)								
	1	..9	10	11	12	13	14	15	16	17	18	19	20	21	22 (C)	23	24	25
A	-	-	-	-	-	-	-	-	-	-	-	-	-	-	-	+8	+32	+32
Ba	-	-	V	-	±	+P	+4	+4	+8	+4	+2	+2	+2	+4	+4	+≥64	+≥64	+256
Bb	-	-	-	-	-	-	-	-	V	V	-	±	+P	+2	+4	+≥64	+≥64	+64

P: Pur   V: Vaccine   C: Challenge

TABLE 4

SEROLOGICAL STUDIES IN GROUP C (MEAN TITRE OF ANTIBODIES)

Group	Born from sow no.	1	2	3	4	5	6	7	8	9	10	11	12	13	14	15	16	17	18	19	20	21	22	23 (C)	24	25	26
Ca	3	+16	+4	+2	+2	+P	+P	+P	+P	V±	-	±	-	-	-	-	-	±	-	-	±	+P	±	+P	+32	+≥64	+128
Ca	4	+32	+16	+4	+8	+4	+4	+2	+2	+2	+2	V+P	+P	+P	+P	±	±	±	±	±	±	±	-	±	+2	+≥64	+128
Cb	3	+32	+8	+4	+4	+2	+2	+P	+P	+P	±	±	-	-	-	-	-	-	-	V	-	±	±	+P +P	+≥64	+≥64	+128
Cb	4	+32	+8	+4	+8	+4	+4	+2	+2	+P	+P	±	±	±	±	±	±	±	±	V	-	±	±	±	+8	+≥64	+128

V: Vaccine   ±: doubtful   +P: + Pur   C: Challenge

The level of antibodies induced by a single vaccination is low in group B; nevertheless the immune system is sensitised. The results of the serological studies in group C are more difficult to analyse.

Table 4 shows that the titre of colostral antibodies fell slowly, but there is a difference between the two litters. The colostral antibodies persisted much longer in the sera of the piglets born from sow 4 than in the sera of those born from sow 3. Indeed, very low titres of antibodies were detected in the sera of the piglets born from sow 4 until the 17th week whereas no antibody was detected after the 12th week in the sera of the litter born from sow 3. It is possible that antibodies can be detected for a much longer period by using more sensitive seroneutralisation techniques. Either no seroconversion, or a very weak seroconversion, was observed in group C. In comparison with group B, it appears clearly that the presence of traces of colostral antibodies interfered with the stimulation of the immune system by the vaccination. It seems that the reaction of the immune system, after challenge, was more intense and rapid in the litter born from sow 3 as if the lower level of colostral antibodies, in comparison with litter 4, allowed a better sensitisation of the immune system by the vaccination. It seems clearer in group Cb.

These observations may explain the differences in the symptoms which appeared after challenge among the group Cb pigs. The clinical signs were more intense in the pigs born from sow 4 than in the litter born from sow 3.

Virological investigations

No virus was recovered from the lungs and the tonsils of the survivors killed 30 to 60 days after inoculation.

DISCUSSION

Several conclusions can be drawn from this experiment. The inactivated virus vaccine provides a protection for fattening pigs against this particular form of AD, but only in the absence of passive immunity. The protection in group B is not complete as slight clinical signs were observed on the inoculated pigs and one pig died after challenge. However, the intensity of the reaction was very weak in comparison with the control group. Moreover, the time necessary for recovering the initial weight was short. It is important to emphasise that only one vaccination was done on the pigs whereas a double vaccination is necessary to provide solid immunity with an inactivated virus vaccine.

It appears, from the results of this experiment, that the presence of maternal antibodies and the level of passive immunity are the main factors which determine the development of an active immunity after vaccination. These results are quite similar to those obtained by Pensaert (1980). However, other factors could influence the intensity of the reaction of the vaccinated pigs after challenge. Indeed, the clinical and pathological observations made in this experiment tend to prove that respiratory disorders are not a result of direct action of ADV especially in view of the nature of the lesions. For example, in the control group, lesions of purulent pneumonia and pleuritis were observed and certainly they are the result of an intense multiplication of bacteria. So, the sanitary status of the pigs before infection with ADV probably has an effect on the intensity of the clinical reactions of the infected animals. ADV affects the pigs as proved by the thermic curve and this severe depression of the pigs' condition favours the onset of a bacterial infection.

In the field, this particular form of AD is often a result of inappropriate measures taken after the onset of the viral infection in a breeding and fattening herd. In most cases, vaccination of the breeders began after the occurrence of the infection (Vannier et al., 1980) and the baconers are not vaccinated. So the virus diffuses throughout the whole herd but passive immunity protects the piglets and the mortality stops in the farrowing house. Generally 'all in-all out' management is not applied in the fattening units of breeding and fattening herds. When 11 - 12 week old piglets are introduced into these units, the maternal immunity is not strong enough to protect them against an ADV infection and they are in contact with older infected pigs which excrete the virus. In these conditions, the infection persists in the fattening units. At the moment, vaccination has no effect on the problem since maternal immunity interferes with the development of active immunity.

In the case of an infection in a non-vaccinated herd, it is possible to prevent trouble in the fattening units by vaccinating all the pigs present on the farm at the time of the onset of the disease. Subsequently, regular vaccination of the sows and pigs is carried out until those pigs born from vaccinated dams arrive in the fattening units (Loquerie et al., 1980). In areas where AD is endemic, systematic vaccination has to be undertaken as a preventative measure in herds which do not sell any breeders.

ACKNOWLEDGEMENTS

The author thanks R. Cariolet for his invaluable assistance and Professor Pensaert who provided the challenge strain.

REFERENCES

Andries, K., Pensaert, M.B. and Vandeputte, J., 1978. Effect of Experimental infection with Pseudorabies (Aujeszky's disease) virus on pigs with maternal immunity from vaccinated sows. Am. J. Vet. Res., 39, 8, 1282-1285.
Loquerie, R. and Ligu, R., 1980. Utilisation d'un vaccin huileux inactivé contre la maladie d'Aujeszky en porcherie infectée. Bilan d'une expérimentation clinique au terme de 5 années. Bull. Soc. Prat. de France, 64, 8, 647-658.
Pensaert, M.B. and Vandeputte, J., 1980. Weight losses in vaccinated fattening swine upon oronasal challenge with Aujeszky's disease virus. Proceedings IPVS Congress, Copenhagen, 118.
Vannier, P., Madec, F. and Tillon, J.P., 1980. The spreading of Aujeszky's disease virus among fattening pigs. Incidence of the virus on respiratory diseases. Proceedings IPVS Congress, Copenhagen, 95.

GENERAL DISCUSSION

P.W. de Leeuw (Netherlands)   There is one point that I would
like to see cleared up and about which there seems to be some
disagreement. How is the infection of cattle performed?
Perhaps I could ask Dr. Biront how he infects his cattle?

P. Biront (Belgium)   Always intranasally. We give the virus
in 10 ml doses, applying 5 ml to each nostril. We use tubes,
the same tube that is used for the IBR vaccine, and the head
is held in a horizontal position.

P.W. de Leeuw   We use the same technique basically. Do you
use this technique, Dr. Wittmann?

G. Wittmann (Federal Republic of Germany)   No, we inject with a
syringe with a long blunt needle.

P.W. de Leeuw   The reason why I am interested in this is that
I still have difficulty in explaining why your animal did not
react the first time when challenged but did react the second
time. Since you have made the experiments, Dr. Biront, I
think you are in a better position to explain this than I am.

P. Biront   I cannot give a satisfactory explanation, I can
only describe what I have seen.

M. Pensaert (Belgium)   I think it is very difficult to reproduce consistently disease in cattle even using high doses,
you must also have luck. Of course, the more virus you use
the better the chance is of achieving infection. But even with
high levels of virus, you do not get a take every time. I do
not know what the factors are that determine whether you get
a take or not, but it is true that using the same dose and the
same animal, one time it will become sick and another time it
will not.

P.W. de Leeuw   If you are that far above the LD_{50} level you would not expect such differences. If you are close to the LD_{50} level I can imagine the situation to be as you say because of all the non specific mechanisms, such as ciliary movement, mucus, that might clear the virus from the nose. However, at high dose levels, even if some of it is washed out, you would expect a certain tolerance.

V. Bitsch   (Denmark)   I agree. If the inoculation dose is not higher than 1 000 units you cannot regularly infect cattle by the respiratory route, especially if it is a virus strain of a low or medium pathogenicity.

P. Biront   I do not think this was the case because this was the virus strain of Professor Pensaert, it kills piglets, gives nervous symptoms, gives pneumonia to fattening pigs etc.

V. Bitsch   Yes, but it is a very low infection dose nevertheless. Our conclusions from investigations of outbreaks in the field are that cattle are not easily infected under natural conditions. I think that this must be the same under experimental conditions. I think we agree, Dr. Pensaert.

M. Pensaert   However, 'why' ; that is another question!

V. Bitsch   It is the same with other animal species apart from swine and possibly sheep.

A. Baskerville   (UK)   I was interested in Dr. Vannier's comments about pneumonia which results from the infection or is superimposed. I think that this is very important to recognise diagnostically. Probably the commonest cause is enzootic pneumonia, which coexists in a large number of herds and can often contribute to the final outcome, as well as Bordetella pneumonia, Pasteurella, Haemophilus and so on. But it is as well to remember that some of the respiratory strains of ADV do in fact cause a pneumonia in their own right, which is extremely extensive; it is necrotising, it is haemorrhagic and animals die of this *per se* . These strains occur in the Far East, in Europe, in Britain and America.

P. Vannier *(France)* We did some virological and bacteriological research on the pigs in this experiment and we could not isolate ADV from the lungs and tonsils of the inoculated pigs killed 30 to 40 days after challenge. However, we did identify bacteria such as *Bordetella, Pasteurella* but no *Mycoplasma*. I think it is an important point that the ADV strain has an effect on the lung. We have a project to inoculate SPF pigs with different ADV strains under very good hygienic conditions and the results will be very interesting. I think it will be very different from the field observations that can be made with these new strains and new forms of ADV. I want to emphasise the effect of bacteria on respiratory disorders of pigs because I am not sure that ADV is the principal cause of these disorders. I think that bacteria are secondary invaders that supervene because of the poor condition of pigs infected with ADV.

V. Bitsch With regard to the pathological changes in the animals that showed pneumonia and pruritus, these changes are exactly those found in *Haemophilus* infections. Did you try to isolate *Haemophilus*?

P. Vannier No, *Haemophilus* is very infrequent in France although it does exist. We could not isolate it from the pigs used in this experiment.

O.C. Straub *(Federal Republic of Germany)* My first question is to Dr. McFerran - why did you leave only two weeks between vaccination and challenge in your experiments?

My second question concerns local immunity after local intranasal immunisation. Would it be feasible to consider when transporting animals from one herd to another, and when vaccinating animals that still have passively acquired antibodies, that you first do an intramuscular (i.m.) vaccination and, at a later stage, a local intranasal one?

194

J.B. McFerran *(UK)* In answer to the first part of that
question I would like to say that two weeks was chosen because
in the fattening units the pigs were starting to develop clinical AD in two to three weeks, so the vaccine had to give
protection in two weeks, otherwise it just wouldn't have
worked.

P.W. de Leeuw We did the vaccination one week after moving
the pigs, if they had to be moved, in order to give them some
time to recover from the transportation stress. You were asking about a combination of intranasal and then intramuscular
vaccinations, is that right?

O.C. Straub *Vice versa.* After transport you have the lower
stress which is the i.m. vaccination, and then when they are
adapted to the place the intranasal vaccination can be given.

P.W. de Leeuw It is difficult to say anything about this
idea since we have not tried it.

Rosalind Gaskell *(UK)* How is your intranasal vaccine attenuated, and does it set up a carrier state itself? Does it
protect against the development of the carrier state following
field virus challenge and what effect does it have when you
vaccinate a pre-existing carrier?

P.W. de Leeuw This is the Bartha strain, the K strain, which
is attenuated. It is the best known strain on the market at
present in the field of live virus vaccines. It is attenuated -
tissue culture attenuated.

Rosalind Gaskell So it is not a temperature-sensitive mutant.
Does it set up a carrier state itself?

P.W. de Leeuw I do not know but this is certainly one of the
things that must be looked into when we carry on our work with
intranasal vaccination.

Rosalind Gaskell   I hesitate to mention another herpes virus,
but with the cat herpes virus we have some evidence to show
that if you vaccinate intranasally you can protect against the
development of a field virus carrier state subsequently, at
least in the short term which may be useful in a field situation. However, this is not quite the same as IBR.

J.B. McFerran   Well, this does reduce the excretion but it
does not stop the field virus becoming established.

P. Vannier   I would like to ask Dr. McFerran about testing the
vaccine. Do you not think that it would be better to vaccinate
the pregnant sows and to challenge the piglets in order to
test passive immunity?

J.B. McFerran   The problem that I have at present is that the
vaccines are now licensed and one is faced with the possibility
of having to test three, four, five batches of vaccine per
year at least, and as more manufacturers come along there will
be more vaccines. From a logistic point of view I do not want
to start to use sows, I want to have very simple tests such as
one has for the attenuated vaccines. What are really going to
be our criteria for saying whether an inactivated vaccine is
a good one or not is the comparison of batches from the same
manufacturer. I certainly do not want to have to go out and
vaccinate 20 pigs and 20 controls and then challenge them every
month!

P. Vannier   Do you think it is a parallel response for testing
passive immunity and active immunity. With AD the most important thing to obtain is passive immunity so if you test only the
active immunity and challenge the piglets, are you sure that
you can extrapolate to the effect that you should have by
vaccinating pregnant sows and challenging the piglet. I understand the practical inconvenience of that, but it can be a
problem to pass on to another test which is different from the
results that we want to obtain in the field.

J.B. McFerran   My problem is not one of trouble in the breeding units; after the initial outbreak the litters live quite happily.   Our problem is with the fattening units.   I think one might say that there might be a case for using a less effective virus on the breeding units.   Listening to some of the discussion, it strikes me that some of the problems are caused by hyperimmunising your sows and getting such high levels of maternal antibody that you then cannot vaccinate your progeny.

P.W. de Leeuw   In the Netherlands, we have had problems with fattening herds for quite some time now.   The problem has switched from breeding to fattening herds.   One of the approaches that we had in mind was to try to hyperimmunise breeding stock in the hope of getting enough maternal immunity to protect the fattening pigs through to the end of the fattening period.   I think that this is an illusion.   Anyway, as it is now it is an illusion - we have to vaccinate these animals when they are on the fattening farm.   And then instead of being an advantage it may become a disadvantage to have very high levels of maternal antibody.   It does depend on the epizootiological situation.

M. Pensaert   Could I ask Dr. McFerran if he has ever tried to vaccinate intranasally with his NIA3 strain?

J.B. McFerran   No, we did do this for the Bartha strain and we got very similar results to those described this afternoon. We did not pursue this because we are not having the problem with pigs with maternal antibody and therefore the slight advantages that the intranasal gave over the intramuscular were not worth the effort in our case.   However, I can certainly see that it might be very useful to get over the problem with maternal antibody.   We have done some preliminary work with maternal antibody, and it does seem that the NIA4 might take better, even given intramuscularly, than the inactivated vaccines.   But this is very preliminary at the moment.   I think certainly that there might still be advantages in the attenuated for the vaccination of pigs with the maternal antibody, even intramuscularly.

M. Pensaert   What kind of virus dose would you recommend?
10^7?

J.B. McFerran   Something like that, it should be fairly high.
I would like to stress though that if we are going to use
attenuated vaccines, we have got to use good ones.

M. Pensaert   You mentioned this morning that this virus does
not show any pathogenicity for rabbits. Did you test this in
other animal species - dogs, cats or cattle?

J.B. McFerran   No, it is very difficult to get licences in
the UK for these animals. I do understand that someone here
has experimented with these animals, at least with dogs. It
was not pathogenic for dogs or for SPF rabbits. Cattle and
sheep have been tested and it was completely non pathogenic
for them.

H. Ludwig   *(Federal Republic of Germany)* I am surprised that there
has been little discussion about alternative types of vaccination. In other fields of herpes virus infections and protection
there are discussions about inactivated vaccines or split vaccines; in IBR infections too. I cannot really understand why,
after such elegant results as those of Dalsgaard on protection,
there are so few movements by others especially those close to
industry. Money can be earned in this way, to produce, for
example, nucleic acid-free protein solutions incorporated in
lysosomes. Instead all discussions seem to be about the live
virus. I think, in the long term, we cannot avoid vaccinating
in the field with highly immunogenic nucleic acid-free material.
If someone was to prove that ADV is really infecting humans,
then things would change rapidly - luckily this is obviously
not the case.

P.W. de Leeuw   I know that there are some groups working on
nucleic acid-free vaccines; they are working on sub-unit
vaccines for example in the USA, but I doubt whether it is
nucleic acid free yet although I do not know how far the work

has progressed. Perhaps someone in the audience here is working on sub-unit vaccines?

H. Ludwig   However, if you use lysates or cut-out arcs or protein mixtures which are centrifuged 100 000 x g, then I think there is less than 0.001% nucleic acid. Instead of that, one is injecting a heavy load of nucleic acid and virus. I think that this should be discussed in much more depth.

J.B. McFerran   I can tell you what is wrong with your suggestion - cost. It is very difficult with the economic situation that pig farmers are in, to produce sub-unit vaccines that pig farmers will use. To produce these vaccines is fine for human use, maybe fine for small animal use but very difficult for pig use.

H. Ludwig   Why for example for small animals?

J.B. McFerran   Because people are prepared to pay for small animals.

P.W. de Leeuw   If you are going to use an inactivated vaccine or a sub-unit vaccine, there must be some plan behind it. Otherwise you cannot expect to eradicate AD or even get it to a lower level, and it will then just cost money. However, I believe the Americans are out to get a vaccine which will give an antibody response they can distinguish from the normal antibody response following a natural infection by some other immunological technique. Then they hope to combine the approach of vaccination with the approach of serologically selecting and removing animals that must be carriers or that have an active infection. It is a combined effort that might well work under some epidemiological circumstances, not ours I'm afraid.

J.B. McFerran   There is a simple way to eradicate using vaccination. If you vaccinate all your breeding animals in the herd you will then reduce the amount of virus being

excreted. You can then select the next generation on serologically negative animals. This works, we have done it.

H. Ludwig   I feel rather doubtful about this since so much
virus is in the country. Nobody has really checked to see how
many latent carriers exist in pig and maybe other herds. We
know that with the IBR system we can activate virus and the
same situation exists with ADV. Even if the animals are not
sick, if you have tested that there is no immune response, and
you think the herd is free, yet after a stress factor, for
example cortisone treatment or perhaps superinfection with
bacteria, the virus will be activated. This is true for all
herpes systems, so why should it be different for AD?

J.B. McFerran   I did not mean that you just do one test, you
must select out the negative pigs and then repeat the test.
Some of these herds are now third or fourth generation. Yes,
it is true that they may still be containing latent virus
which one day will break, but three or four generations really
isn't bad.

A. Baskerville   There are two possible ways of distinguishing
between vaccinal and field antibody. One is by the simple
inclusion in the vaccine of a unique protein such as keyhole
limpet haemocyanin. At a small additional cost on the vaccine,
this would act as a unique marker so that those pigs would then
have antibody to KLH, whereas obviously those in a field
infection would not.

Another approach that would probably be even more
simple would be an ELISA test based on classes of antibody like
IgM, IgG. This would probably separate these two, although
such a system has not yet been worked out but I feel it is an
area that could be very fruitful.

Another point about the vaccination methods - I do not
think that we should forget the oral route because this is
extremely important with live vaccine, as for other vaccines
in other species. If you accept the fact that it is generally
assumed that a large proportion of immunocompetent cells which

are stimulated in the gut will home to mucous surfaces, then, if the gut is stimulated and immunised you can get quite good immunity at the nasal mucosa as a result. I believe that live vaccine given orally, which is much easier with pigs than the intranasal method, is one approach that could be used.

P.W. de Leeuw   I am not sure whether your last suggestion has really been proven. Going back to your suggestion of adding something to the vaccine, this concept depends also on the chance to make enough viral antigen and then getting legislation through to allow you to carry on if you do find positives. For example, if this is done the vaccine will have to be limited to one or two that are likely to be used. You must first show your results to be such that the legislators will support your ideas. This is a major problem in itself.

K. Dalsgaard *(Denmark)*   I am afraid that when talking about markers in inactivated vaccine that one of the available vaccines has already a relatively harmful marker. I do not know whether you are aware of this and I would like your comments on the fact that at least one of the inactivated vaccines against AD is based on IBRS-2 cells reported to be persistently infected with classical swine fever virus.

P.W. de Leeuw   Yes, I am aware of that. We have checked it in the first 10 or 20 animals that we vaccinated with the vaccine that is produced on IBRS-2. I believe, Dr. Terpstra, that you checked the blood group production of the cells.

C. Terpstra *(Netherlands)*   Yes, that's right. We have tested some sera from a herd which we knew how many times the sows had been vaccinated and revaccinated. We have not been able to demonstrate this but I must state that we have used the conventional neutralisation test and I understand that at Lindholm a more sensitive test has been used to demonstrate this. They have also demonstrated the antibodies against swine fever in animals that had been vaccinated at a short interval.

The normal interval for vaccination in sows is 6 or 12 months. We have not been able to demonstrate this with our techniques.

P. Vannier I have a comment to make about this since we did the same test as Dr. Terpstra on a large number of sera with this type of vaccine and we never found any antibodies against swine fever.

M. Pensaert Considering the results given in Dr. Terpstra's paper in relation to the MK25, I was wondering if Dr. van Oirschot had an explanation for his early effect, considering that Dr. Terpstra did not find the virus at all after four days of vaccination? Have you any explanation for the mechanism of your earlier effect? You said that even 2 days after vaccination they have already some kind of protection.

J. Th. van Oirschot (Netherlands) There is a certain degree of protection even two days after vaccination with that modified live vaccine. I do not have a very good explanation for how the immune mechanisms work, but I assume that the quick, secondary immune response plays an important role in that early protection.

M. Pensaert Two days is certainly quick for a secondary immune response.

J. Th. van Oirschot It is quick but when you remember the figure of the neutralising antibodies, you can see a difference on day 7 after challenge. The titres in the pigs vaccinated two days before challenge were higher than in the controls. This is not perhaps a real secondary immune response when you compare it to the other two groups but there is something going on two days after vaccination.

M. Pensaert But it certainly is not an interference, as earlier suggested.

J. Th. van Oirschot   We could not detect interferon but that
is not to say there was not any interferon because we used
secondary pig kidney cells for detecting interferon. Some
people say that they used the Madin-Darby bovine kidney cells
which are more sensitive in detecting porcine interferon than
secondary pig kidney cells. So if we had used the Madin-Darby
bovine kidney cells we might have been able to detect interferon.

T. Terpstra   This is an additional comment to the question of
Dr. Pensaert. The fact that we did not find the MK25 virus
after four days in the tissues that are normally examined for
diagnostic purposes at *post mortem* does not mean that there
might not have been virus in some other part of the body. This
should not be forgotten.

M. Pensaert   It has to be somewhere!

SESSION V

LATENT INFECTION

Chairman: G. Wittmann

DETECTION OF AUJESZKY'S DISEASE VIRUS AND VIRAL
DNA IN TISSUES OF LATENTLY INFECTED PIGS

H.-J. Rziha, P.C. Döller and G. Wittmann

Federal Research Institute for Animal Virus Diseases,
D-7400 Tübingen, Federal Republic of Germany.

ABSTRACT

   *Different organ tissues of latently infected pigs were investigated
for the presence of Aujeszky's disease virus (ADV) and viral DNA. As
indicated by the failure to detect infectious virus, latency was established
beyond 7 weeks post infection (p.i.). After immunosuppression, however,
latent virus was readily reactivated. By in situ cytohybridisations and
DNA - DNA reassociation kinetics, the presence of viral DNA was demonstrated
in neural tissues during the latent state.*

INTRODUCTION

   A major characteristic of the herpesviruses is their
ability to establish latent infections. It is also known that
Aujeszky's disease virus (ADV) persists in the infected host.
Frequently, upon primary infection, the virus remains in the
recovered host, even though neutralising antibodies have been
developed. Infectious virus cannot be demonstrated, and no
clinical symptoms are seen. However, reactivation of the latent
virus occurs readily after various endogenous and exogenous
stimulations. As a consequence, infectious virus will be produced leading to the recurrence of the disease (Baringer, 1975;
Stevens, 1978). Therefore, the latently infected host must be
considered as a virus carrier, and as a potent source for
spreading the virus. It is well established that human herpesviruses can persist in sensory ganglia in an inactivated state
(Galloway et al., 1979; Puga et al., 1978; Sequiera et al.,
1979). An unresolved question is which kinds of mechanism
determine and regulate the phenomenon of latency and reactivation.
   The objective of our studies was to determine more precisely
the range of tissues supporting a latent ADV infection, and
the cell types that harbour the latent virus.

MATERIALS AND METHODS

   Ten-weeks old pigs were infected intranasally with 10^9

G. Wittmann, S.A. Hall (eds), Aujeszky's Disease. ISBN-13:978-94-009-7555-2

TCID$_{50}$ of the virulent ADV strain Phylaxia. Various organs,
the mucous membrane of the nose, and neural tissues were
removed from the animals during the acute and latent state of
the infection. To reactivate latent ADV, the pigs were immuno-
suppressed for 3 - 4 days with prednisolon (1 250 mg/animal).

The presence of infectious virus in the single organ
tissues was demonstrated by cocultivation and tissue fragment
culture methods on BHK- and MDBK cells, respectively.

Molecular hybridisation techniques were applied for the
detection of ADV-DNA or RNA. The method of *in situ* cytohybridisation (Moar and Klein, 1978) permits the localisation of viral
DNA in cells or tissues. Frozen thin sections are fixed on
coverslips, and the cellular DNA is denatured *in situ* by alkali
without severe disruption of the cyto-architecture. Purified,
in vitro radioactively labelled ADV-DNA or complementary RNA
(cRNA), is applied to the treated cells under annealing
conditions for about 20 hours. Non-hybridised labelled ADV-DNA
or cRNA is washed away, and the hybrid molecules formed are
scored by autoradiography and Giemsa-staining of the cells.

For the determination of the amount of ADV-DNA in latently
infected cells, DNA-DNA hybridisation in solution was performed
for measuring the reassociation kinetics (Huang and Pagano,
1977). Cellular DNA extracted from different organ tissues and
radioactively labelled ADV-DNA, both made single-stranded and
fragmented, are mixed, and incubated under annealing conditions.
The double-stranded DNA molecules formed are separated after
varying incubation times from the non-hybridised DNA single
strands by hydroxylapatite chromatography. The formation of the
hybrid DNA molecules follows a second order kinetic depending
upon the concentration of the viral DNA sequences present. As
compared to the negative control reaction, the annealing rate
accelerates with increasing amounts of viral DNA, and the number
of viral genome-equivalents per cell can be calculated.

RESULTS AND DISCUSSION

Beyond 7 weeks p.i. regularly latency was established,
as no infectious virus could be detected. Latent ADV, however,
was readily reactivated up to 64 weeks p.i. following immuno-

suppression (Table 1). After endonuclease digestion the DNA
fragment pattern of the reactivated virus was identical to
that of the inoculated virus.

TABLE 1
REACTIVATION OF ADV FROM LATENTLY INFECTED PIGS AFTER IMMUNOSUPPRESSION

Organ tissues	Weeks p.i.						
	11	12	13	16	26	32	64
Tonsils	3/4[a]	1/2	1/2	1/2	2/2	2/2	2/2
Lymphnodes	2/4	1/2	1/2	0/2	2/2	2/2	NT[b]
Lungs	3/4	0/2	NT	2/2	2/2	2/2	NT
Mucous membrane	2/4	1/2	NT	NT	2/2	2/2	NT
Brain	NT	2/2	1/1	1/2	2/2	2/2	1/2
Olfactorial bulb	1/1	1/1	0/1	NT	2/2	2/2	1/2
Medulla	1/1	2/2	1/2	NT	2/2	2/2	0/2
Trigeminal ganglia	NT	1/1	NT	NT	2/2	2/2	0/2
Spinal cord	NT	2/2	NT	1/2	2/2	2/2	NT

a) Number of positives/number of animals tested.
b) Not tested.

TABLE 2
DETECTION OF ADV-DNA IN DIFFERENT ORGAN TISSUES

Organ tissues	1	1.5	4	5	6	7	11	13
Tonsils	+	+	+	+	+	-	-	-
Lymphnodes	+	+		+	+	+	-	-
Lungs	+	+		+	+	-	-	
Brain				+		+	+	
Olfactorial bulb						+	+	
Vagus nerve						+	+	
Maxillar nerve						+	+	
Trigeminal ganglia							+	+
Spinal cord						+	+	

During the acute state of infection, ADV-DNA was readily detectable by *in situ* cytohybridisation in tonsils, lungs and lymphnodes. In virus free animals 5 and 6 weeks p.i. the same organ tissues were shown to contain only small amounts of ADV-DNA. Similarly, small amounts were demonstrated in the lymph-nodes of one pig (Figure 1). Table 2 summarises our present results of the *in situ* hybridisations of organ tissues of acutely and latently infected, non-immunosuppressed animals.

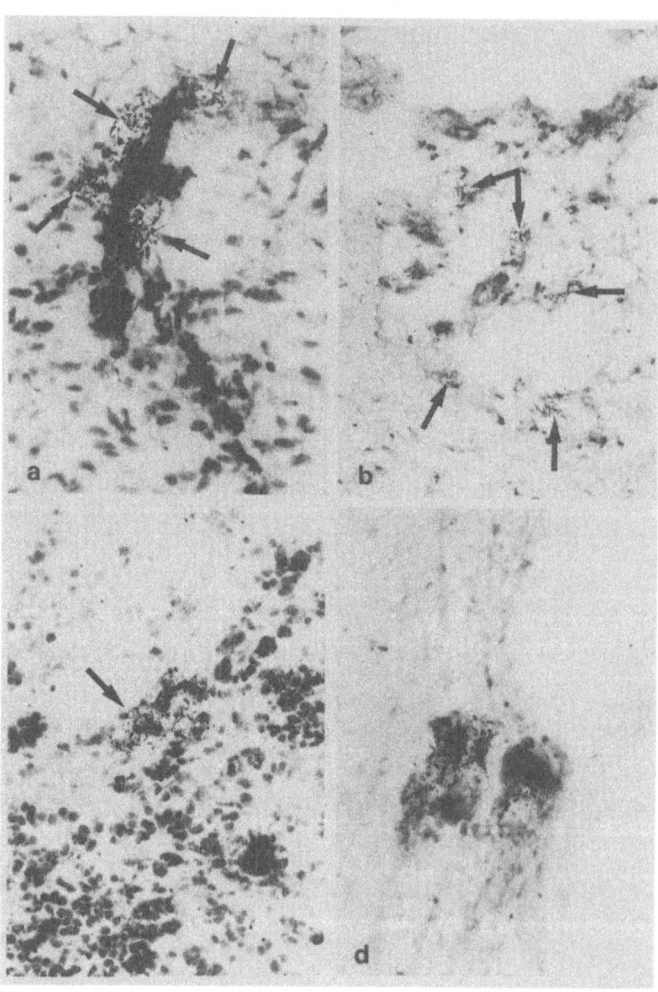

Fig. 1. Detection of ADV-DNA (arrows) by *in situ* hybridisation with
^{3}H-labelled ADV-DNA (8×10^6 cpm/µg) to frozen sections of vagus
nerve 7 weeks p.i. (a and b), lymphnodes (c), and tonsils (d),
5 weeks p.i., respectively.

It is remarkable that in the latent state viral DNA was preferentially formed in the neural tissues. This might indicate the presence of latent ADV in ganglia and cells of the central nervous system, as suggested by other workers, (Huang and Pagano, 1977) in contrast to those organs, where the main virus production occurred during an acute infection. Further experiments are in progress to confirm these findings.

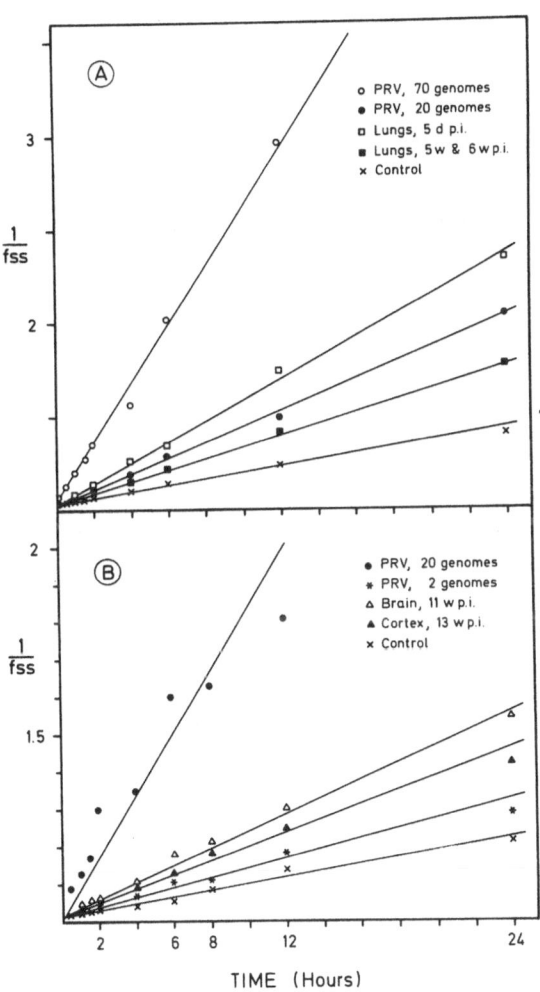

Fig. 2. Reassociation kinetics of ^{32}P-labelled ADV-DNA (3×10^7 cpm/µg) with different organ cell DNAs. Hybridisation was performed in 0.3 M NaCl at 70°C. fss = fraction remained single-stranded.

To determine the amount of the ADV genome in latently infected cells, we used the method of the DNA-DNA hybridisation in solution for measuring the reassociation kinetics. Thus, we were able to calculate the amount of ADV-DNA sequences in lungs 5 and 6 weeks p.i. at a level of 15 genome equivalents per cell, and 30 genomes/cell in lungs 5 days p.i. (Figure 2A). In the brain and cortex of latently infected animals 11 and 13 weeks p.i. about 5 and 6 genomes/cell were found, respectively.

Finally, for detection of a possible transcriptional activity of the latent ADV-DNA, we have begun to examine some latently infected tissues for the presence of virus-specific RNA by *in situ* hybridisations. Initial, very preliminary, results might indicate the occurrence of PRV-mRNA in neural tissues of pigs 13 weeks p.i. However, more detailed studies need to be made to reproduce and confirm these findings.

REFERENCES

Baringer, J.D., 1975. Herpes simplex virus infection of nervous tissue in animals and man. Progr. Med. Virol. 20, 1-26.
Galloway, D.A., Fenoglio, C., Shevehuk, M. and McDougall, J.K., 1979. Detection of herpes simplex RNA in human sensory ganglia. Virology 95, 265-268.
Gutekunst, D.E., 1979. Latent pseudorabies virus infection in swine detected by RNA-DNA hybridization. Am. J. Vet. Res. 40, 1568-1572.
Gutekunst, D.E., Pirtle, E.C., Miller, L.D. and Stewart, W.C., 1980. Isolation of pseudorabies virus from trigeminal ganglia of a latently infected sow. Am. J. Vet. Res. 41, 1315-1316.
Huang, E.-S. and Pagano, J.S., 1977. Nucleic acid hybridization technology and detection of proviral genomes. In 'Methods in Virology' (Ed. K. Maramorosch and H. Koprowski) Academic Press, New York and London. Vol. 6, 457-497.
Moar, M.H. and Klein, G., 1978. Detection of Epstein-Barr virus (EBV) DNA sequences using *in situ* hybridization. Biochim. Biophys. Acta 519, 49-64.
Puga, A., Rosenthal, J.D., Openshaw, H. and Notkins, A.L., 1978. Herpes simplex virus DNA and mRNA sequences in acutely and chronically infected trigeminal ganglia of mice. Virology 89, 102-111.
Sequiera, L.W., Carrasco, L.H., Curry, A., Jennings, L.C., Lord, M.A. and Sutton, R.N.P., 1979. Detection of herpes simplex viral genome in brain tissue. Lancet 2, 609-612.
Stevens, J.G., 1978. Latent characteristics of selected herpesviruses. In 'Adv. Cancer Res.' (Ed. G. Klein and S. Weinhouse). Academic Press, New York - San Francisco - London. Vol. 26, 227-256.

OCCURRENCE OF CLINICAL AUJESZKY'S DISEASE IN IMMUNOSUPPRESSED LATENTLY INFECTED PIGS

G. Wittmann, H.-J. Rziha and P.C. Döller

Federal Research Institute for Animal Virus Diseases
D-7400 Tübingen, Federal Republic of Germany.

ABSTRACT

Latent Aujeszky's disease virus (ADV) infection in pigs could be reactivated by the application of high doses of prednisolon 9½ months after infection. The animals showed clinical signs of illness and shed ADV in their nasal secretion.

INTRODUCTION

It is well established, as we heard from the last speaker, that Aujeszky's disease virus (ADV) causes a persistent infection in pigs. However, almost nothing is known about the clinical reactivation of the latent infection, since the animals are usually killed shortly after immunosuppression to obtain material for virus isolation. Davies and Beran (1980) reported that ADV was spontaneously shed in the nasal secretion of a sow after parturition 19 months post infection. However, this sow did not show clinical signs of AD.

MATERIALS AND METHODS

Five pigs aged 12 months, which had recovered from experimental ADV infection 9½ months previously, were treated with high doses of prednisolon. We injected 1 875 mg of the drug on each of 4 consecutive days. The temperature and the clinical state were monitored continuously and nasal swabs were taken daily. The washing fluids of the swabs were inoculated in tenfold dilutions into BHK cell culture tubes for infectivity titration. The animals were killed between day 29 and 33 after immunosuppression. Ground tissue suspensions of nasal mucosa, tonsils, retropharyngeal lymphnodes, lung, bulbus, brain stem, medulla, spinal cord, spleen, kidney and inguinal lymphnodes were inoculated in tenfold dilutions into BHK cell culture tubes for ADV isolation. In addition, cocultivation of the minced tissue in MDBK cell monolayers was performed.

G. Wittmann, S.A. Hall (eds), Aujeszky's Disease. ISBN-13:978-94-009-7555-2

212

The sera of the animals were examined at certain intervals by the neutralisation test. This test was also used to identify the ADV isolates from the nasal swabs. The test was performed in the presence of 10% guinea pig complement according to the method previously described (Wittmann et al., 1976; Jakubik and Wittmann, 1979).

RESULTS

Figure 1 shows the mean values of fever, nasal virus excretion in TCD_{50} per swab and neutralising titres (ND_{50}). At the beginning of the treatment the animals had ND_{50} titres between 1 : 169 and 1 : 294. During the treatment there was no significant decline in antibody titres. On day 5 their titres ranged between 1 : 223 and 1 : 512 (mean 1 : 309). On day 8 an insignificant decrease had occurred with 2 of the 5 animals and the titres range was between 1 : 97 and 1 : 294 (mean 1 : 192). On day 11 the range was between 1 : 223 and 1 : 384 (mean 1 : 284). Thereafter, there was an increase in titres.

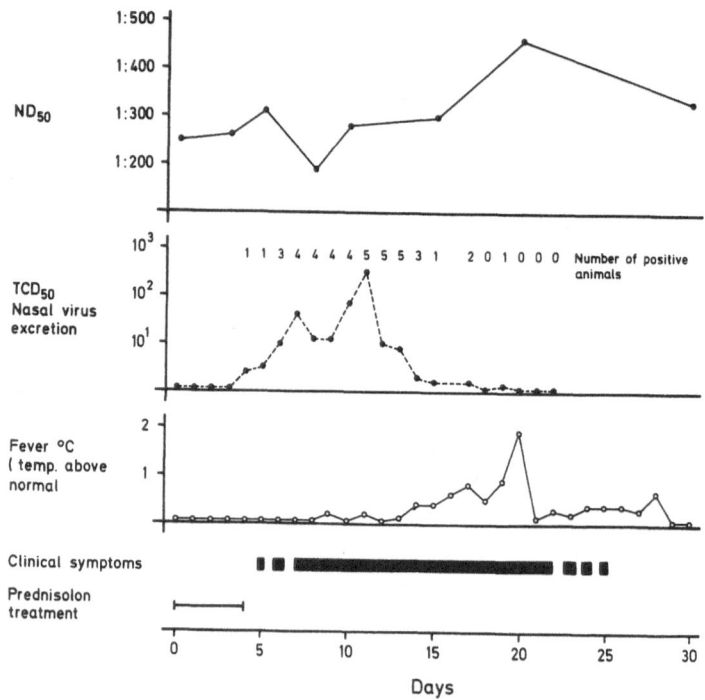

Fig. 1.

Before immunosuppression the pigs were very lively. However, between days 5 and 7 after immunosuppression the animals became very quiet and apathetic. Strong salivation and nasal discharge appeared. The mouths were covered with foam. There was loss of appetite and the animals lay down most of the time. Three of the pigs lost their voices. A rise in temperature of at least 0.5°C above the normal level began between days 13 and 19 after immunosuppression. It lasted minimally one day and maximally 7 days. With every animal the peak of fever was reached on day 20, with a rise in temperature between 1.2°C and 2.4°C above the normal level. The first signs of recovery were seen on day 23. The animals, except one with pneumonia, had recovered by day 26.

ADV could be isolated from the nasal secretions of all the animals. The first appearance of virus varied between day 4 and day 11 after the beginning of the prednisolon treatment. The period of virus excretion lasted minimally 3 days and maximally 14 days. The maximal virus titres found with the animals were between $10^{2.1}$ and $10^{3.5}$ TCD_{50} per swab. Identification of the excreted virus was made by neutralisation.

The ND_{50} values of the sera were between 1 : 389 and 1 : 512 (mean 1 : 463) on day 19. Compared with the initial ND_{50} titres there was an increase between 1.7- and 3-fold, indicating that ADV multiplication had occurred. The animals were killed between days 29 and 33. No ADV could be isolated directly from the different tissues and organs. However, ADV could be isolated from the central nervous system and from the lungs of 2 of the 5 animals by cocultivation. Examination by biochemical methods (see Rhiza et al., in this Proceedings) has not yet been made. Uninfected control pigs which were treated with prednisolon showed no signs of illness, no fever and no cytopathic agents in the nasal swabs.

Thus it was demonstrated that a latent persistent ADV infection can be activated by stress to such a degree that clinical manifestation occurs. We do not know if such a strong stress as we used is very common in nature. However, we think that under very unfavourable conditions it may be possible.

REFERENCES

Davies, E.B. and Beran, G.W., 1980. Spontaneous shedding of pseudorabies
    virus from a clinically recovered post parturient sow. Am. J. Vet.
    Med. Ass. 176, 1345-1347.
Jakubik, J. and Wittman, G., 1979. Neutralizing antibody titres in pig
    serum after revaccination with an inactivated Aujeszky's disease
    virus (ADV) vaccine. Zbl. Vet. Med. B, 325, 741-751.
Wittman, G., Bartenbach, G. and Jakubik, J., 1976. Cell-mediated immunity
    in Aujeszky's disease virus infected pigs. Arch. Virol. 50, 215-222.

GENERAL DISCUSSION

<u>J. Asso</u> *(France)* I would like to know the control used with fluorescent antibodies?

<u>H.-J. Rziha</u> *(Federal Republic of Germany)* I have not done this because there is only a small chance of obtaining positive results.

<u>P. Vannier</u> *(France)* Do you think that pigs latently infected for a long time could possibly have no antibodies in the serum?

<u>G. Wittmann</u> *(Federal Republic of Germany)* Up to the present we have tested pigs up to 15 months after infection and we have always found neutralising antibodies in differing degrees, sometimes 1 in 4, sometimes 1 in 6, sometimes 1 in 50 or 1 in 60.

<u>P. Vannier</u> By using conventional methods?

<u>G. Wittmann</u> We use complement neutralisation tests by the addition of complement.

<u>A. Baskerville</u> *(UK)* What is your feeling, Professor Wittmann, about the percentage of animals which become latently infected? I am not clear whether people are implying that a high proportion of naturally infected pigs become latent carriers or whether this is a very small proportion. Do your experiments shed any light on this?

<u>G. Wittmann</u> We did not test pigs from the field but only used our pigs that were infected with high doses of virus. We tested up to the present from d.p.i. 7 to 15 months after infection. We have tested about 20 animals and from these about 10 were between 6 months and 15 months after infection and in every case we could find infective virus after immunosuppression and in some instances after co-cultivation of the nervous tissue with BHK cells, for example. I think that if an animal is infected by ADV it is almost certain to become a latently infected animal.

<u>A. Baskerville</u> You think that is the normal state of affairs?

<u>G. Wittmann</u> Yes, I believe so.

J. Th. van Oirschot *(Netherlands)* Dr. Rziha, do you have some
data on the sensitivity of your viral hybridisation *in situ* test
in comparison with normal cultivation techniques?

Secondly, are you sure you used viral strain Phylaxia
because there could perhaps be some strain differences in producing latent infections?

H.-J. Rziha Perhaps so, but we have inoculated with the strain
Phylaxia and so I used the same viral DNA for detection. The
sensitivity of the *in situ* hybridisation is much more sensitive
than co-cultivation methods. It is much more sensitive than
pre-association kinetics because only small amounts of viral
DNA can be detected clustered in some single cells in the overall range of cells. However, this is a difficult technique and
we have to perform many experiments to reproduce such results.
It is a very sensitive technique.

J. Th. van Oirschot How many sections do you have to examine
before you can make a slide such as you have shown here?

H.-J. Rziha You have to do many controls and if in the controls
there is a high background then you can forget the experiments.

Rosalind Gaskell *(UK)* I would again like to make a comment on
the cat herpes, which is in many ways similar. You get a latent
infection in the majority of animals and easy reactivation with
corticosteroids. I would like to make a suggestion, Professor
Wittman, that you try rehousing stress to see if this can stimulate episodic secretion. In the cat, 15% of cats will shed
virus following rehousing stress, whereas with corticosteroid
the figure is more like 60%. Obviously these animals are more
likely to be the ones that are epidemiologically important in
that they shed under natural stress conditions. Again in the
cat, there seems to be a spontaneous shedding rate of about 1%.

H. Ludwig *(Federal Republic of Germany)* In the IBR system similar
experiments have been performed and, as Dr. Gaskell says, it is
very common in herpesviruses.

Dr. Wittmann, did you ever try to superinfect those latent
infected swine and did you check on the resulting virus? I am
not sure if in the pig that strain which is latent could be

blocking another infection, but if this is so a vaccine could easily be devised which would make the state of latency and a further virulent infection would be blocked. Or did you check for the DNA pattern?

H.-J. Rziha In some cases and not in others. In some cases I have checked the reactivated virus after DNA cleavage with two or three different enzymes. In all cases the DNA pattern was identical with the inoculated strain of Phylaxia.

G. Wittmann In completing our results, I would like to mention that we also tried to isolate ADV from vaccinated pigs after infection. Three and six and a half months after infection we could find virus without immunosuppression, by co-cultivation in tonsils, lungs and brain. After immunosuppression the virus could be isolated directly from the brain, the nasal mucosa, the tonsils and the spinal cord with titres between $10^{2.1}$ and $10^{4.3}$ TCD_{50}. This shows that after infection with ADV, vaccinated immune pigs will also become latently infected.

Sheila Cartwright (UK) This is not directly related to the papers presented this morning, but I was wondering if anyone had any evidence that piglets from a sow infected in utero have been born as virus shedders? Is there any evidence of an autoimmunity system working? Has anyone here done any work along these lines?

H. Ludwig I would like to make a parallel comment. Some years ago Dr. Storz in the department at Ciccscn, working with an IBR system, was able regularly to isolate from 20 normal bovine foetuses 20% IBR virus. It came from bovine foetal spleen cells. So I would suggest that if someone carefully co-cultivates embryonic spleen cells or perhaps lymphoid cells he might activate the virus. Perhaps Dr. Gaskell has tried this with cats.

Rosalind Gaskell In the cat, the situation appears to be slightly different in that the virus appears to be confined more to the upper respiratory tract and we have not detected placental transmission in kittens born to latently infected carrier queens.

Sheila Cartwright It is certainly fairly common in the field to recover virus from dead piglets following transplacental

infection. I am thinking more of the parvo virus story when
you not only get it from the dead or mummified piglet but also
from the live piglet. You can quite easily isolate the virus
from this animal. If this did happen in AD you would have your
natural shedder all the time.

O.C. Straub *(Federal Republic of Germany)* Dr. Ludwig's comment requires another comment as far as Dr. Storz's examinations are
concerned because the phenomenon that he found at Giessen he
tried to find elsewhere too. He did not succeed; he tried in the
USA and in other parts of Germany and so I believe that normally
foetuses are not latently infected by IBR. In general IBR virus
causes an abortion and I think the same will be true for ADV.
I might add in comparing IBR and ADV and prednisolone treatment
that you cannot use as high a dose in cattle as Dr. Wittmann
used in pigs. That level was extraordinarily high and it is
also remarkable that the white blood picture hardly changed.
The white blood picture for the hog hardly changes while for a
bovine it changes dramatically after administration of such a
high amount of corticosteroids.

H. Ludwig I would like to make a comment to that comment! I
think that until it is tested it remains unproven. Everyone
knows that these herpesviruses are integrating. They are even
probably integrating in the genome or are covalently linked to
the genome. Many of the human herpesviruses are found in lymphocytes and there is a good parallel with the IBR system in that
Porter in California, using normal mink which had been fed with
contaminated meat, could isolate from spleens and activate IBR
virus.

I think that these herpesviruses and most probably AD
viruses have an affinity with the lymphoid system and if you
treat this lymphoid system at the right stage of development
then you can activate. The foetus might have it at a stage when
it is not activated and it might stay there or even go vertic-
ally.

The phenomenon at Giessen was repeated 10 years ago.
Maybe there is a strain which preferentially integrates.

J. Th. van Oirschot Dr. Wittmann, have you ever tried to establish latency in maternally immune pigs because theoretically
this could be a method to create latent carriers without the
development of neutralising antibodies?

G. Wittmann No, I have not done this. The experiments would be
very time and space consuming. It would be impossible to take
up all the accommodation at the Institute for my pigs!

Rosalind Gaskell Again a comment on the cat, because I think it
has some parallels. Yes, we established a latent infection in
kittens which were protected by maternal antibody; they did not
show any clinical signs and they then became seronegative. Subsequently, they were reactivated with corticosteroid and then
they developed antibody following the reactivation of latent
virus.

If I may make another comment about Dr. Ludwig's comment,
I would dispute that all herpesviruses are latent in connection
with a lymphoid tissue because there are the simply neurotropic
latent herpesviruses, for example, herpes simplex virus, where
lymphoid tissue does not seem to be particularly important in
latency.

SESSION VI

EPIDEMIOLOGY, CONTROL AND ERADICATION

Chairman: J.B. Andersen

DANISH LEGISLATIVE MEASURES FOR THE CONTROL OF AUJESZKY'S DISEASE

J.B. Andersen

Danish Veterinary Services,
Frederiksgade 21, DK-1265 Copenhagen K, Denmark.

ABSTRACT

For the control of Aujeszky's disease (AD) under Danish conditions, infection control seems preferable to disease control. An efficient diagnostic technique is available, the elite breeding system (comprising about 20 000 breeding sows) and the AI system (covering about 20% of the services) is free from the disease, and the Danish geography facilitates movement control and the establishment of regional control programmes. The boar stations have been ruled by legislation including AD control since 1970, and AD has, since April 1980, been subject to general legislation worked out in accordance with Danish experience and tradition for control and eradication of contagious diseases in domestic animals. In February 1981 the first regional control programme was implemented for the island of Bornholm.

INTRODUCTION

The control of infectious diseases in domestic animals can be carried out according to two main principles, disease control and infection control. The two principles can be used separately or in combination. The decision as to which system will be preferable depends on the nature of the infectious agent, the efficiency of current diagnostic methods and the prevalence of the infection. For viral infections vaccination will be a main factor in disease control programmes. However, unlimited and uncontrolled vaccination will make infection control programmes difficult or impossible, as it is not possible for the time being to distinguish between antibodies from vaccination or from infection. The complete eradication of an infectious disease from the national herd will in the final phases at least, demand a pure infection control programme.

Experience indicates that Aujeszky's disease (AD) may be controlled in the Danish national herd by using an infection control programme, which in the beginning could be combined with disease control in the form of a limited and strictly controlled vaccination. The main reasons for this assumption are the following: a) The development of a highly sensitive

G. Wittmann, S.A. Hall (eds), Aujeszky's Disease. ISBN-13:978-94-009-7555-2

virus-serum neutralisation test has improved and facilitated
the testing procedure (Bitsch and Eskildsen, 1976; Bitsch, 1980);
b) a voluntary control programme implemented in 1967 in the
elite breeding herds has ensured that the elite breeding herds
and the candidate elite breeding herds comprising about
20 000 breeding sows have been kept free from AD (Bitsch, 1980;
Borgen et al., 1969); c) the AI system has been ruled by legislation since 1970 and is free from AD; d) the geographical
division of Denmark into well separated regions facilitates
movement control and regional control programmes, as demonstrated
in previous national control and eradication campaigns e.g. the
brucellosis campaign (Wøldike Nielsen, 1955) and the leukosis
campaign (Flensburg and Streyffert, 1977).

LEGISLATION

Boar stations

The boar stations, which for the moment cover about 20%
of the services, have been ruled by legislation since 1970.
Boars to be used for artificial insemination must pass a
1 month quarantine before entering the boar station. At the
end of the quarantine period before being released they must
among other examinations pass a virus-neutralising antibody
(VNA) test for AD. AI boars are routinely retested at least
every second year for AD.

The Aujeszky's Disease Order

Since 1980 AD has been subject to general legislation
by the Aujeszky's Disease Order issued by the Ministry of
Agriculture, April 16, 1980. A brief survey of this order
is given below:
1)   AD is made a notifiable disease.
2)   AD shall be suspected to exist in a herd:
   a)   if piglets below 3 weeks of age exhibit convulsions
        and/or paralysis succeeded by a high mortality rate,
        or
   b)   if convulsions and/or paralysis associated with

intensive localised pruritus occur in one or more
animals.

3)   A herd shall be considered infected by AD when the presence of virus or specific antibodies has been confirmed
in samples from the herd.

4)   A herd shall be considered free from AD when all sows,
boars, gilts and any swine not born and reared in the
herd have passed a serological examination. Free herds
must be retested at least every second year (15% of the
breeding animals), and only swine from other free herds
are allowed to be introduced.

5)   A certificate can be issued for animals from a free herd.

6)   Vaccination can only take place with permission granted
and on conditions issued by the Veterinary Services.

7)   Natural mating of swine in other ownership is restricted
to the present level and the present establishments.

The order is worked out in accordance with Danish
experience and tradition for eradication of contagious diseases
in domestic animals e.g. tuberculosis (Tønnesen, 1971) and
brucellosis (Wøldike Nielsen, 1955). The fight against the
disease is primarily implemented as a voluntary programme to be
carried out in co-operation with the pig producers with the
emphasis on buying and selling pigs accompanied by a certificate
stating freedom from AD. The test scheme for the free herds is
similar to the scheme which has proved efficient in connection
with the use of the P_{24}^{37}-VNA test in elite breeding herds
(Bitsch, 1980). Vaccination has so far not been carried out.

Regional control programmes

The next step will be the implementation of more
restrictive regional control programmes, and the first has
already been put into force for the island of Bornholm. AD
has never been diagnosed on this island, and a screening examination of all sows and boars slaughtered during a 3 week
period in September 1980 (555 samples) showed no positive
reactions. This investigation has been followed by a monitoring programme, according to which all boars at the island
must be tested serologically when being slaughtered, and live

pigs can only be moved to the island after permission from the
Veterinary Services in accordance with the Order concerning
movement of live swine to Bornholm, issued by the Ministry of
Agriculture, February 5, 1981.

Screening examinations and control measures for pigs
being moved into a region are being planned for other parts of
the country. In these cases it is also foreseen that establishment of movement control could be necessary within the region.

REFERENCES

Bitsch, V., 1980. The application of a highly sensitive virus-serum
    neutralisation test in screening examinations of large numbers of
    swine sera for antibody to Aujeszky's disease virus. Proc. Congr.
    Int. Pig Vet. Soc.,Copenhagen, 101.
Bitsch, V. and Eskildsen, M., 1976. A comparative examination of swine
    sera for antibody to Aujeszky virus with the conventional and a
    modified virus-serum neutralization test and a modified direct
    complement fixation test. Acta. Vet. Scand., 17, 142-152.
Borgen, H.C., Bitsch, V. and Bendixen, H.J., 1969. Aujeszky's sygdom hos
    svin i Danmark - forekomst og forholdsregler 1964-1969. Medlbl.
    danske Dyrlægeforen., 52, 995-1006.
Flensburg, J.C. and Streyffert, B., 1977. The control of bovine leukosis
    in Denmark. Nord. Vet.-Med., 29, 49-67.
Tønnesen, J.J., 1971. Bekæmpelse af kvægtuberkulose i Jylland. Diss.
    (A/S Carl Fr. Mortensen, Copenhagen).
Wøldike Nielsen, F., 1955. Brucellosis control and eradication in Denmark.
    Vet. Rec., 67, 939.

ON THE EPIDEMIOLOGY OF AUJESZKY'S DISEASE IN DENMARK AND THE POSSIBILITIES OF ITS CONTROL

V. Bitsch[1] and J.B. Andersen[2]

[1]State Veterinary Serum Laboratory, Bülowsvej 27, DK-1870 Copenhagen V, Denmark.

[2]Danish Veterinary Services, Frederiksgade 21, DK-1265 Copenhagen K, Denmark.

ABSTRACT

The most prominent epidemiological features of Aujeszky's disease (AD) related to its occurrence in Denmark are described. The annual number of outbreaks diagnosed in pig herds in recent years has been relatively low, i.e. 60 to 85. Syncytia-forming isolates of the virus seem to possess a generally higher pathogenicity for swine and cattle than non-syncytia-forming strains. Syncytia-forming strains of the virus were isolated from about 20% of outbreaks in pig herds in 1978 and 1979, but from 50% of outbreaks in 1980. These outbreaks predominantly occurred in the western and northern parts of Jutland. Outbreaks caused by syncytia-forming virus strains have occurred in a number of closed herds, and it is concluded that in some such cases there was evidence to support the notion of an air-borne transmission of the virus. Central parts of the pig breeding system are free from AD. The herds concerned are controlled serologically and are not allowed to have contact with animals from uncontrolled herds. With the present limited occurrence of AD the possibility of air-borne herd-to-herd transmission of virus is not considered to be a hindrance which will render a complete eradication of the infection impossible, but it is stressed with regard to this that the control and eradication of AD in big herds should receive special attention.

INTRODUCTION

Aujeszky's disease (AD) has occurred in cattle in Denmark since 1931, and has been recognised as a disease entity in pigs as from 1964. In the present paper the most important epidemiological features of this infection are described, and the possibilities of its control and eradication are discussed.

THE PREVALENCE OF THE INFECTION

Table 1 gives the number of outbreaks diagnosed by isolation of virus in the different animal species, apart from swine, since 1964. The annual number of outbreaks in pig herds in the various parts of the country is shown in graph form in Figure 1.

From earlier investigations (Borgen et al., 1969) it was concluded that infected animals would be found in about every

228

TABLE 1

VIROLOGICALLY CONFIRMED OUTBREAKS OF AUJESZKY'S DISEASE IN ANIMALS OTHER
THAN SWINE

	1964	65	66	67	68	69	70	71	72	73	.74	75	76	77	78	79	80
Cattle	6	9	13	9	10	9	8	9	16	13	17	12	12	10	8	9	8
Dogs	–	–	–	2	5	8	10	6	3	3	2	2	–	–	1	2	5
Cats	–	–	–	1	1	2	–	–	–	–	–	–	–	–	–	–	1
Farm foxes	–	–	–	–	2	–	–	–	–	–	–	–	–	–	–	–	–
Red foxes	–	–	–	1	4	3	6	2	2	4	4	3	3	2	5	5	4
Other species	–	–	1[1]	–	–	–	–	1[2]	–	–	–	–	–	–	1[3]	–	1[4]

[1]: sheep;   [2]: badger;   [3]: goat;   [4]: captive roe deer.

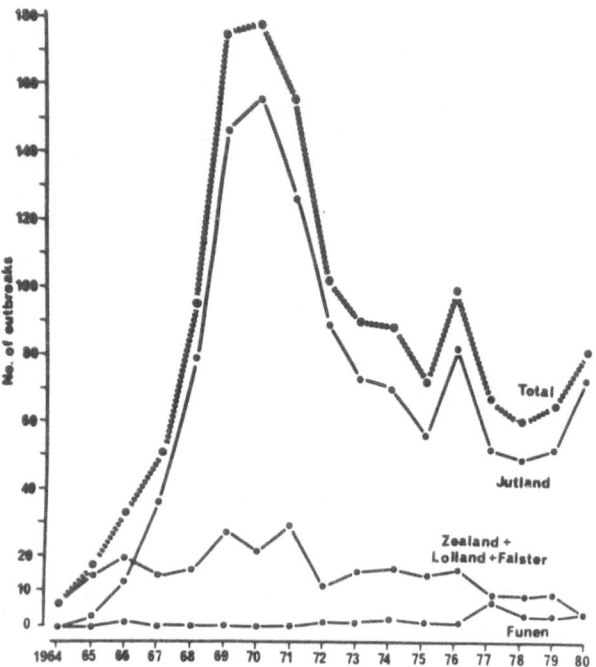

Fig. 1.   Virologically confirmed outbreaks of Aujeszky's disease 1964 - 1980
in pig herds from different parts of the country.

third non-closed pig herd in Zealand and Jutland. (Closed herd: in this context herds where only contacts with animals from AD-controlled herds are accepted.)

Before 1970 nearly all herds were non-closed, but today the situation is different. More than 50% of breeding sows are found in rather big herds (Table 2), and nearly all these herds are closed. In a recent limited examination of herds from a certain area in Western Jutland, infected animals were found in 3 of 6 non-closed herds as against 1 of 19 closed herds (Christensen and Bitsch, 1980). These findings together with other results demonstrate that AD in infected parts of the country will be frequently found in non-closed herds, but is not likely to be encountered in closed herds.

TABLE 2

INFORMATION ABOUT PIG HERDS IN DENMARK.

I. Number of herds and sows	
Breeding herds without fattening pigs:	25 000
Breeding herds with fattening pigs:	28 000
Herds with fattening pigs alone:	20 000
Number of sows:	1 000 000

II. Size of herds

1 to 9 sows:	52% of herds,	with 11% of all sows
10 to 29 sows:	29% of herds,	with 25% of all sows
over 29 sows:	19% of herds,	with 64% of all sows

III. Elite breeding herds

330 herds with 15 000 breeding animals

IV. SPF herds

1 560 herds with 94 000 sows; 900 000 pigs slaughtered annually. 9% of all sows, 8% of all slaughter pigs, and 2% of herds are SPF.

V. Artificial insemination

450 000 first inseminations are performed annually

About 20% of all sows are inseminated

Reference: National Committee for Pig Breeding, 1980.

230

PATHOGENICITY OF VIRUS STRAINS

From a study on the differences in pathogenicity among
strains of Aujeszky's disease virus (ADV) it was concluded that
strains which were highly pathogenic for swine and cattle would
regularly cause syncytia formation in tissue cultures, in contrast to strains of lower pathogenicity, which would be non-
syncytia-forming (Bitsch, 1980b).

About 50% of the isolates from outbreaks in 1980 have
been found to be syncytia-forming, as against 20% in 1978 and
1979. This indicates that a change in the disease situation
has occurred. The localisation of the herds from which syncytia-
forming and non-syncytia-forming strains were isolated are
shown in Figures 2a and 2b, respectively. Seven isolates were
not evaluated. The figures illustrate that the syncytia-forming
virus strains are predominantly found in Western and Northern
Jutland.

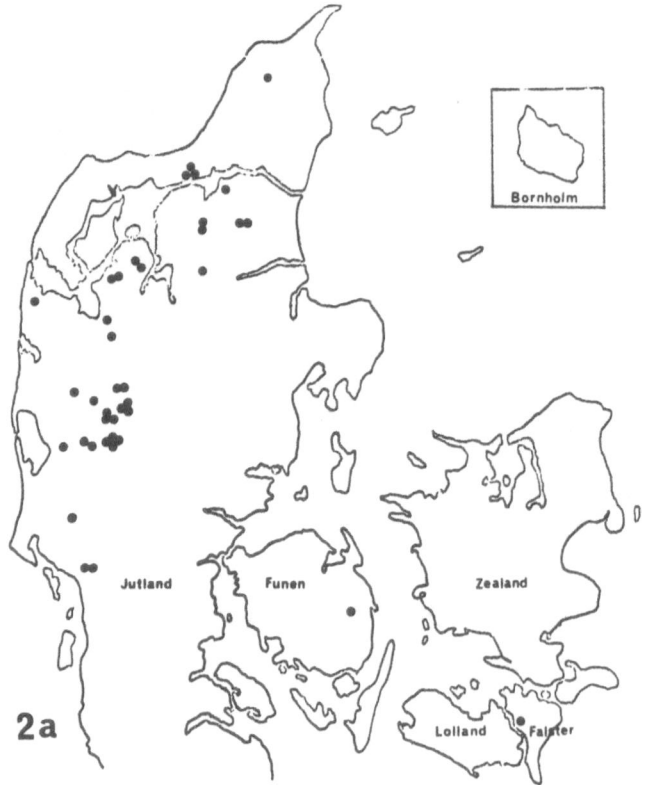

Fig. 2a. The localisation of pig herds with outbreaks of Aujeszky's disease
in 1980 caused by syncytia-forming virus strains.

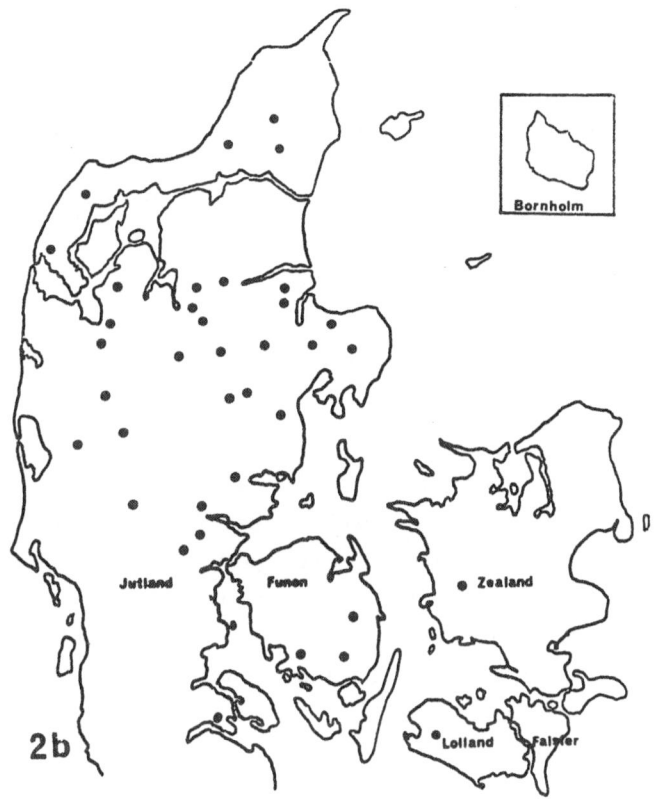

Fig. 2b   The localisation of pig herds with outbreaks of Aujeszky's disease
in 1980 caused by non-syncytia-forming virus strains.

HERD-TO-HERD TRANSMISSION OF THE INFECTION

      Evidence of a transmission of the infection by man from
one herd to another has been found in a very few cases,
especially where virus was transferred to cattle (Bitsch, 1975a,
b, c). But still, until recently, the main conclusion was that
herds got infected because of contacts with pigs shedding virus
during the acute infection phase or during a later period after
reactivation of the infection (cf. Bitsch, 1974).

      After the appearance of highly pathogenic strains of the
virus, however, this general point of view can no longer be
strictly maintained. Outbreaks caused by syncytia-forming virus
strains have occurred in herds where no immediate contact with
animals from infected herds was imaginable. In each of the

small clusters of infected herds in Western Jutland shown in
Figure 2a, the infection appeared in the individual herds within a relatively short period. Several of them were closed, and
in each group the herds were situated not more than 2 km, and
most often less than 1 km, from each other. This would seem to
point to a common origin of the infection for the herds in each
group.

Two possible explanations of the introduction of the
infection in such cases were conceivable: either transmission
by rodents or airborne herd-to-herd spread of the virus.

Rodents

The question was whether infection with especially
syncytia-forming virus strains could be established in a mouse
or rat population. In experiments with young mice infected
nasally, the inoculated animals regularly died, while in-
contact mice survived and were susceptible to challenge infection. Similar results were obtained with young rats. When
relatively low virus doses were used, some rats survived, but
they did not resist subsequent challenge infection. In one
cage, brain and chest organs of a dead infected rat were eaten
by 2 in-contact animals, and one of these died 4 days later.
The conclusions were the same for both syncytia-forming and
non-syncytia-forming strains: mice and rats were susceptible
and would die, if they were infected, but the infection was
not easily established. The results did not seem to support
the idea of a herd-to-herd spread of the infection by rodents.
These findings are consistent with those obtained by others
(Kirkpatrick et al., 1980).

Airborne transmission

In cases of respiratory infection in cattle it has often
been found that virus has been carried from swine to cattle
within a herd over a distance of 10 - 20 m because of air
currents produced by ventilators. Some such cases have been
reported previously (Bitsch, 1975b), and another example is
shown in Figure 3. In this particular case there were no pigs

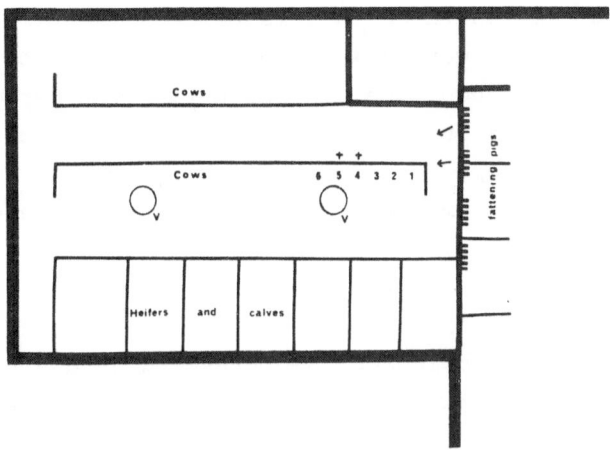

Fig. 3. Plan of a cowhouse, where Aujeszky's disease occurred in two cows
(4 and 5) showing anterior localisation of pruritus, which is indicative of respiratory infection. Arrows illustrate air currents
from the room with fattening pigs through two windows with broken
panes.

in the cow house. The two affected cows were placed close to
a ventilator and were infected by the respiratory route: one
showed pruritus on its head, the other licked its shoulder
vigorously, and virus was isolated from the lungs of the latter
animal. It was evident that they had inhaled virus from the
fattening pigs in the room next to the cow house.

This illustrates the fact that ventilators in a pig house
with an acutely infected herd will blow considerable amounts of
virus out into the open air. It is difficult to estimate the
risk of an airborne herd-to-herd transmission, but logically it
will depend on the efficiency of the ventilation system, the
size of both the infected and the uninfected herd, weather
conditions, and the characteristics of the virus strain. Two
examples of probable airborne transmission of strains of high
pathogenicity are described in the following.

(1) An SPF herd was infected about 6 months after it had
been established. Buildings were new, and food was in special
containers. Presence of mice or rats had not been observed,
and introduction of the infection by persons seemed unlikely.
AD had been diagnosed some years previously in a herd with over

700 sows and 3 000 fattening pigs situated just 500 m away.
A number of blood samples taken in this herd at the time of
outbreak in the SPF herd were all found to be serologically
positive. Information about the weather during the period
immediately prior to the outbreak did not exclude the possibility of an airborne spread from the previously infected herd.
In fact, considering the amounts of virus that would be produced by 3 000 acutely infected fattening pigs the risk of an
airborne transmission to neighbouring herds may appear to be
overwhelming.

(2) AD was diagnosed in a closed breeding herd with over
200 sows, which all appeared to become clinically affected.
Approximately three weeks earlier, an outbreak had started in a
herd 125 m away with 150 sows and 200 fattening pigs. Wind
directions during the acute outbreak in this herd would support
an airborne transmission to the closed herd.

It is noteworthy that the infection in the above cases,
as well as in some other cases where an airborne transmission
seemed likely, was considered to have been spread from herds
with fattening pigs.

Finally it should be mentioned that if virus of high
pathogenicity is shed from infected pigs in higher amounts than
virus of low pathogenicity (which seems reasonable), airborne
herd-to-herd transmission would lead to predominant occurrence
of highly pathogenic strains in big herds.

POSSIBILITIES OF INFECTION CONTROL

Application of AD vaccines cannot prevent the spreading
of field virus, so vaccination will not be dealt with here.

For the control of the presence of AD in pigs it is
important to employ a test that is sensitive enough to detect
all infected animals. The modifications of the virus-serum
neutralisation test used in Denmark (Bitsch and Eskildsen,
1976; Bitsch, 1980a) seem to fulfil this requirement, although
a short quarantine or isolation period prior to the sampling
will be necessary in some cases.

Elite breeding herds, AI boar stations and the central
SPF breeding herds are already controlled and free from AD, and

all SPF herds (Table 2) are considered to be free (Andersen, these proceedings). For these herds, as well as for others that want to maintain their freedom from infection, it is essential to avoid contacts with animals from uncontrolled herds.

The main problems associated with an eradication programme extended to comprise all herds in a part of the country are that many pig breeders will be reluctant to comply with the requirement to close the herds, and also that the infection can be transmitted even to closed herds under certain conditions. However, the fact that the infection has so far been diagnosed in only 4 out of 1 560 SPF herds, and not at all for many years in elite breeding herds, indicates that airborne transmission is still not a factor which will decisively impede the possibilities of complete eradication. On the other hand, it must be realised that the method of implementation of an eradication programme may have to be somewhat different in areas where syncytia-forming virus strains are prevalent.

From the circumstances that the economic importance of the infection is chiefly connected with its occurrence in big herds, and that large infected herds in particular constitute a risk of infection for neighbouring herds, it follows that the control and eradication of the virus in big herds should receive special attention.

Virus strains of low pathogenicity seem to predominate in relatively small non-closed herds, where the sows are served naturally by boars from boar centres. It is likely, however, that if natural service were replaced by artificial insemination, the infection would disappear from a high proportion of the herds in the course of a few years.

REFERENCES

Bitsch, V., 1974. La maladie d'Aujeszky au Danemark. Cah. Méd. Vét., 43 211-219.
Bitsch, V., 1975a, b, c. A study of outbreaks of Aujeszky's disease in cattle. I. Virological and epidemiological findings. II. Further investigations on the routes of infection. III. Selected outbreaks of a special interest regarding epidemiology. Acta vet. scand. 16, 420-433, 434-448, 449-455.

Bitsch, V. and Eskildsen, M., 1976. A comparative examination of swine sera for antibody to Aujeszky virus with the conventional and a modified virus-serum neutralization test and a modified direct complement fixation test. Acta vet. scand., 17, 142-152.

Bitsch, V., 1980a. The application of a highly sensitive virus-serum neutralization test in screening examinations of large numbers of swine sera for antibody to Aujeszky's disease virus. Proc. Congr. Int. Pig Vet. Soc., Copenhagen, 101.

Bitsch, V., 1980b. Correlation between the pathogenicity of field strains of Aujeszky's disease virus and their ability to cause cell fusion - syncytia-formation - in cell cultures. Acta vet. scand., 21, 708-710.

Borgen, H.C., Bitsch, V. and Bendixen, H.J., 1969. Aujeszky's sygdom hos svin i Danmark. Forekomst og forholdsregler 1964-1969. Medlbl. danske Dyrlægforen. 52, 995-1006.

Christensen, G. and Bitsch, V., 1980. Undersøgelse over forekomsten af Aujeszky's sygdom i udvalgte konventionelle sobesætninger i en vestjydsk egn. Dansk Vet. Tidsskr. 63, 954-955.

Kirkpatrick, C.M., Kanitz, C.L. and McCrocklin, S.M., 1980. Possible role of wild mammals in transmission of pseudorabies to swine. J. Wildlife Dis. 16, 601-614.

EPIDEMIOLOGY AND CONTROL OF AUJESZKY'S DISEASE
IN GREAT BRITAIN

Sheila Cartwright

Central Veterinary Laboratory,
Weybridge, Surrey, UK.

ABSTRACT

A brief history of Aujeszky's Disease (AD) in Great Britain is given, together with a description of the current situation, including the results of a recent serological survey of 25 000 sera. The probable methods of spread of the disease in a small endemic area in East Anglia are examined, including wildlife studies and finally current Ministerial policy and possible methods of control of the disease are examined.

HISTORY

Aujeszky's disease (AD) was not described in England until 1953 (Done and Venn, 1953) although it had been reported from Northern Ireland as early as 1939 (Lamont and Shanks, 1939). Prior to 1973, AD was really of little concern to the pig industry in this country; the number of cases confirmed yearly were of the order 1 to 5 and were spread throughout England with no cases being recorded in Scotland and very few in Wales. Examination of over 5 000 sera collected from pork and bacon weight pigs in England, Scotland and Wales between 1958 and 1961 showed below 1.0% to contain antibodies to ADV. Several surveys were carried out by the UK Ministry of Agriculture, Fisheries and Food (MAFF) in the 1960s and 1970s and were negative showing there was little or no subclinical disease in the country.

In 1973 the number of infected premises detected increased to double figures for the first time, the increase being mainly confined to the east side of the country where the pig population is at its densest. During the following five years the number of new infected premises recorded each year rose to between 15 and 20, still not a vast number by comparison to some other European countries but definite foci of infection were becoming established both in East Anglia and Yorkshire and serum surveys and detailed field investigations bore out the fact that in a certain area of Suffolk the disease was becoming

G. Wittmann, S.A. Hall (eds), Aujeszky's Disease. ISBN-13:978-94-009-7555-2

endemic. In the West Country the clinical signs of the
disease were not so obvious and infected premises were often
detected through investigations of reproductive failure or by
deaths in hounds due to the feeding of infected pig meat. In
this area the pig farms are well distributed and there are also
large fattening units receiving pigs from many parts of the
country.

In the years 1979 and 1980 the number of new infected
premises detected yearly was of the order of 30 - 35, many of
these being concentrated in the small area in Suffolk. During
1979 - 80, 25 567 sera were examined from 3 045 premises;
these comprised eight separate surveys including the annual
surveys of the 260 Elite herds (members of either the MAFF
sponsored Pig Health Scheme or of the Pig Health Control
Association), where only one new reactor herd was found. Fat
pigs surveyed at abattoirs showed little rise in the percentage
of reactors over the past years. Only 7 infected premises
were detected of which 3 were known positive herds and one had
purchased animals from a known positive source. Sampling of
breeding stock from farms in endemic areas revealed 5 new
infected premises. It would therefore seem that the number
of unrecorded outbreaks of disease in England is still at a
very low level.

The type of disease seen, with a few exceptions, has
altered little over the years, with nervous disease in very
young piglets often leading to a high mortality, and dullness
and anorexia in older animals combined with reproductive
failure in breeding sows and gilts. Few signs of respiratory
disease as described by Baskerville (1971) with strain NIA2,
were recorded. Indeed the only consistent difference in
clinical signs that we could detect was a very mild disease
with a low mortality in baby piglets which had been imported
from Northern Ireland via breeding gilts. As cases were
traced across the country due to this source, the severity of
the disease remained at the same low level and similar results
were obtained following experimental infection of piglets with
this isolate. Two Pig Health Scheme Herds found to be serologically positive have never shown clinical signs of the

disease despite repeated investigations and were subsequently cleared by culling the reactors. Clinical disease in fattening houses due to AD appeared to be minimal and was often confined to just a mild anorexia.

EPIDEMIOLOGY

A closer look was taken at a small endemic area in Suffolk to try and explain some of the 'spread factors' in order to see what could be recommended for control of the disease.

Size of the unit

It is an accepted fact that this plays an important role and we have found that in the majority of small herds of less than 50 breeding sows that the disease has been more or less self limiting. This has been borne out by successive visits and serum sampling of such herds.

Area density

The number of units situated in a certain area plays a definite role in the rate of spread. This is again borne out by the situation which has developed in this particular area where the pig units are very closely associated and also the situation which developed in certain areas in Holland where the density of pig units was very high.

Stocking density

This factor combined with the number of air changes per hour seems to be related to the rapidity of spread of a disease within a house.

The movement of the pig

Unlimited evidence has been put forward to show that this is one of the most important ways of spreading AD around the country and when the animal is a latent carrier the disease may not manifest itself on the new premises for many months.

Field evidence has shown delays of up to 20 months. However in this particular study little of the lateral spread of the disease was traced to the movement of stock.

Movement of objects

The movement of farm vehicles, delivery lorries, shared equipment etc. Strong circumstantial evidence was often found for this but nothing was proven. Many farms now have isolated loading bays but not all and it certainly seems to be one of the most common breakdown points in disease security.

We have found no evidence for spread by slurry - the method of storage would surely not encourage survival of this virus. Workers in Northern Ireland and USA have apparently succeeded in isolating AD virus from faecal material. Despite repeated efforts we have not been successful although we have isolated AD virus from the wall of the ileum following experimental infection.

Man himself

Man could be of considerable importance purely as a mechanical vector. No well documented evidence exists as regards active infection of the human species. We have examined at least 12 sera from people in close contact with ADV with negative results. Even as a passive vector it is again only circumstantial evidence, as nasal swabs and fingernail scrapings taken from workers on infected premises and at the laboratory have been negative. However in close-knit communities such as the one under investigation it would seem a very likely factor.

Movement of other species

Birds

Laboratory experiments at Weybridge have produced no evidence to suggest that birds act as anything other than mechanical vectors in the spread of AD. Following intranasal instillation of AD virus and the feeding of virus infected material to 12 starlings we failed to isolate virus from excreted material nor did the birds seroconvert, as tissues taken at *post mortem* were negative.

Birds are probably considerably involved in local spread mainly by the transfer of infected material from area to area i.e. from the manure heap to the feeding area and in the case of the larger carrion eaters by the removal of dead piglets or aborted material.

Insects

This is another species that may be involved in the local spread of AD. At Weybridge investigations into the possible involvement of cockroaches showed that the virus did not persist or survive in this species.

Small mammals

Mammals such as rats, mice, voles, shrews etc., have been trapped on known infected premises and in endemic areas but no isolations of AD virus have been made or neutralising antibodies detected in sera. Two reports were received of sick rats having been seen on infected premises but no material was sent for examination. Wildlife experts consider that rats occupying pig premises would be too well fed to move far from the locality. Certainly recent evidence (Maes et al., 1979) has been produced to show that brown rats could be involved in localised spread by consuming infected material and then infecting food with their oro-nasal secretions but the fact that they might be long term carriers of the virus has been discounted.

Larger mammals

We have examined material from over 50 foxes and badgers trapped and found dead in endemic areas. Virus has been recovered from the brain and spinal cord of a fox found dead on an infected premises. There was also evidence of pruritus and at *post mortem* the stomach contents showed evidence of the animal having been in the habit of consuming piglet material. No further recoveries have been made from foxes trapped on the same premises so there is no evidence of spread from fox to fox. Two foxes were also found dead near another infected farm but no material was submitted. A recent paper (Kirk-patrick et al., 1980) described the findings of examining 73 wild and domestic mammals trapped in an area endemic for AD in the USA, with virus recoveries made from 16. Laboratory experiments showed that the racoon could be infected by association with infected pigs or consuming infected material and vice versa but no evidence could be produced to show transmission from racoon to racoon. A similar situation possibly exists with the fox and thus on a fox's normal rounds nearby premises could become infected.

A similar situation exists with cats and dogs. The interval between infection and death in cats is given as 3 - 7 days (Hagemoser, 1980). We have made many isolations of virus from cats found dead or dying on infected pig premises. Since 1973 36 dogs have been shown to have died of AD in this country, 27 of these were from 4 packs of hounds who were subsequently shown to have been fed on infected pig meat and the remaining 9 were from known infected premises.

These species could be involved over a fairly short period of time in local spread of infection.

Wind dispersal

This is a further factor to be seriously considered in an area of dense pig population. In Suffolk the direction of the gradual spread of the disease over the years from village to village is that of the prevailing wind. Certainly the output of virus from a densely populated, highly infected, fattening unit must be considerable and deserves further attention.

From these observations we have learnt little that is new and which can be of use to a pig farmer in an endemic area and can do little other than to advise greater disease security as regards transport lorries, visitors, rodent control, discouragement of scavengers from feeding areas with consider-able emphasis being placed on greater farm hygiene i.e. disposal of carcases, aborted material etc., and burning of any infected bedding. A possible investigation into windborne infection is also being considered. Despite these recommendations for disease security 3 herds which were within this area and in which the disease was eradicated - by serological testing and culling (two) and by slaughter and repopulation (one) - became reinfected within the year, whereas those outside the area where the disease had been eradicated by similar means, have remained clear.

Policy and control

Field observations on the control of the disease by eradication have been carried out on a limited scale. We have successfully cleaned up 6 - 7 herds by serological testing and culling. In the seventh there was continuing disease in a large fattening house on the same premises which acted as a continuous source for reinfection. As already mentioned two of the farms were in an endemic area and subsequently became reinfected.

We have also investigated the situation of depopulation and restocking and the type of disinfection required and the length of the interim period with successful results.

Aujeszky's Disease became a notifiable disease in Great Britain under The Aujeszky's Disease of Swine Order in August 1979. All clinical disease suspected as AD must be reported to the Ministry of Agriculture, Fisheries and Food (MAFF) and standstill regulations apply until a visit has been made by a Ministry veterinarian. Advice is given but no restrictions are kept in force following confirmation of the disease except in the case of Pig Health Scheme herds.

Following discussions with the industry, a recent poll of pig producers was held by sending out a questionnaire from MAFF to determine the degree of support for an eradication scheme which would be financed by a levy on all pig producers. The total response received was well below that of the agreed 75% and it has therefore been agreed to proceed no further with arrangements for a levy scheme and MAFF will continue its discussions on future action with the industry.

The most likely options to be taken up are those of strongly encouraging the continued freedom from AD of the 260 Elite herds and promoting purchase of breeding stock from these herds, keeping the disease notifiable, and controlling the disease situation by a) herd eradication by serological testing and culling and/or b) vaccination with possible constraints on usage.

At present there is no vaccine licensed for use in Great Britain although with the changing situation in Northern Ireland similar action would probably follow in this country.

REFERENCES

Baskerville, A., 1971. Res. Vet. Sci., 12, 590-592.
Done, J.T. and Venn, J.A., 1953. Unpublished work.
Kirkpatrick, C.M., Kanitz, C.L. and McCrocklin, S.M., 1980. J. Wildlife Dis., 16, 601-614.
Maes, R.K., Kanitz, C.L. and Gustafson, D.P., 1979. Am. J. Vet. Res., 40, 393.
Hagermoser, W.A., Hill, H.T. and Kluge, P., 1980. Proceedings IVPS Congress Copenhagen, 96.

EPIDEMIOLOGY AND CONTROL OF AUJESZKY'S DISEASE IN THE REPUBLIC OF IRELAND

P. Lenihan and P.J. O'Connor

Veterinary Research Laboratory,
Abbotstown, Castleknock, Co. Dublin, Ireland.

ABSTRACT

The relationship between Aujeszky's disease and changes in the pattern of pig production in the Republic of Ireland is discussed. The emergence of Aujeszky's disease in the 1970s as a serious economic problem was associated with the establishment of large intensive units. Eighty primary cases of disease were diagnosed between 1973 and 1980, more than half of these occurring in herds ranging in size between 100 - 1 700 sows. All zoosanitary measures failed to halt the advance of Aujeszky's disease and, in addition, serological surveys indicated that subclinical infection was widespread.

In Ireland the first recorded isolation of Aujeszky's disease virus (ADV) from swine was from two litters of pigs in Northern Ireland in 1939 (Lamont and Shanks). Even though this was the first confirmed case there is strong evidence on clinical grounds that the disease existed in the pig population long before that time.

Subsequently, Lamont (1964) reported 23 separate cases involving deaths in cattle, sheep, pigs, dogs and a cat. Since then, the disease has been described on different occasions both in Northern Ireland (Gordon and Luke, 1955; McFerran and Dow, 1964) and in the Republic of Ireland (McErlean, 1960).

In the Republic the disease is primarily one of pigs and other species are rarely affected. Prior to the early 1970s the disease was only occasionally diagnosed in the field and in the laboratory. Even accepting that some cases were undiagnosed, the disease was of little importance. This was related to the fact that the greater proportion of the national sow herd was dispersed in thousands of smallholdings with the average number of sows per holding being very small. This system of sow rearing afforded Aujeszky's disease (AD) little opportunity to develop as a serious problem. When the virus gained entry to a small sow herd the mortality was invariably low and the disease was to a large degree self limiting.

G. Wittmann, S.A. Hall (eds), Aujeszky's Disease. ISBN-13:978-94-009-7555-2

Not a single case of AD was diagnosed in fattening herds during this period even though some 20% of all fattening pigs were produced in large intensive units. These varied in size from 1 000 - 8 000 pig fattening places and were stocked by recruiting weaner pigs from the numerous producers in the respective catchment areas.

Beginning in the mid 1960s the traditional sow rearing systems underwent radical changes and the pattern of pig production altered appreciably (Table 1). There emerged a new generation of pig producers who availed themselves of financial incentives to invest heavily in buildings and stock. In the period between 1965 - 1979, there was a sixfold reduction in the total number of farms engaged in sow rearing. By 1979, 81% of the national breeding herd was located in some 800 units, whilst the remaining 19% of sows were dispersed in 7 200 farms (Table 2).

TABLE 1

CHANGES IN THE STRUCTURE OF THE NATIONAL PIG HERD 1965 - 1979

Year	1965	1975	1979
Holdings with pigs	89 734	23 000	10 200
Pigs per holding	13	38.3	109.9

TABLE 2

CHANGES IN THE STRUCTURE OF THE NATIONAL SOW HERD 1965 - 1979

Year	1965	1975	1979
Holdings with sows	48 205	16 900	8 000
Holdings with 20 sows or more	376	700	800
Sows in 20 + holdings %	9.9	54.1	81.4

Considerable restructuring of the fattening herds occurred concurrently to accommodate the changes which were taking place in the breeding herds. This resulted in the establishment of

many new fattening herds, some of which were attached to breeding herds.

In 1973 the first serious outbreak of AD was diagnosed in
a large unit. This outbreak heralded an absolute change in the
epizootiology of AD in Ireland resulting in serious neonatal
mortality and varying incidences of abortion and infertility.

Eighty primary outbreaks of AD occurred between 1973 and
1980 (Figure 1). This does not include secondary outbreaks in
herds where the disease was previously diagnosed. Of these, 42
cases involved herds which ranged in size between 100 - 1 700
sows. In herds of this size the virus is likely to become
enzootic. Therefore it is not unreasonable to suppose that a
cumulative total of approximately 16 000 sows, in these 42 herds,
are potentially infected - representing some 13% of the national
sow population.

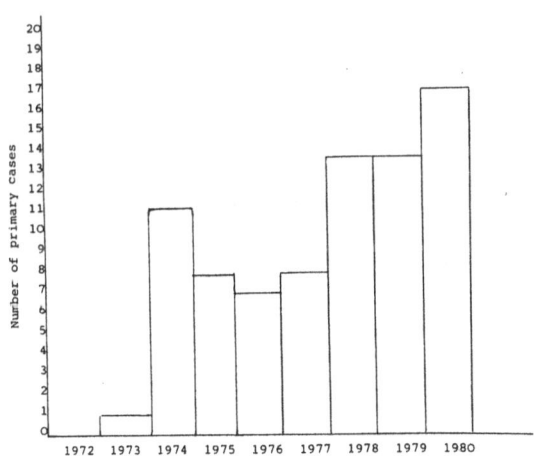

Fig. 1. Incidence of Aujeszky's disease in the Republic of Ireland since
         1972.

The origin of infection could in some instances be
directly related to the introduction of carrier breeding stock
from infected breeding herds. However, in most instances the
source of infection was not determined.

Compared with breeding herds the disease in fattening units to date has been less important. It has tended to occur sporadically and its appearance seems to be related to some stress factor such as changes in feed or temperature fluctuations. Morbidity can be variable but mortality is generally low. In 1973 there was one exception to this pattern of disease when a serious problem arose in a large fattening herd. A virulent virus producing high mortality with respiratory involvement was isolated. The disease has subsequently recurred on a few occasions in this herd with far fewer losses.

During 1974 a serological survey for ADV was carried out in both fattening pigs and sows. The test used was the serum neutralisation test at a ½ dilution of serum, performed in microplates as described by Rosenbaum et al. (1972). The sera were obtained from a large bacon factory in the Leinster area. Every effort was made to sample pigs from as many different farm sources as possible.

Twenty-four percent of sows had ADV antibodies whereas only 0.5% of fattening pigs were positive (Table 3). This result indicates that a sizeable proportion of sows, unlike the fattening pigs, had been exposed to ADV. These results are similar to those reported by McFerran et al. (1966) when it was found that 27% of sows had antibody but only 3 bacon-weight pigs out of 575 tested were positive.

TABLE 3

AUJESZKY'S DISEASE SURVEY 1974 - SERA FROM SOWS AND FATTENING PIGS

	Number of sera	SN titre 1/2	% positive 1/2
Sows	829	196	23.6
Fattening pigs	200	1	0.5

In 1978 another survey for AD was carried out on sera from fattening pigs (Table 4). These sera were collected on this occasion from 123 farms which were geographically widely distributed throughout the country. All these herds were known to be clinically free from AD. The sera were screened at a ½ dilution. Four percent of the pigs on this occasion had ADV antibody which was a significant increase on the 1974 survey.

By the late 1970s there was ample evidence of both clinical and sub-clinical AD in the country. Furthermore, it was reasonable to assume that the disease had become enzootic in the majority of large infected units. Support for this thesis is shown by the persistence of high antibody titres in five large herds (Table 5).

TABLE 4

AUJESZKY'S DISEASE SURVEY 1978 - SERA FROM 123 FATTENING HERDS

Number of sera	SN titre 1/2	% positive 1/2
1 108	45	4.0

TABLE 5

SERA FROM 5 LARGE INFECTED BREEDING HERDS

Herd	Number of sera	Interval between initial isolation of AD virus and sampling	SN titre $\geq 1/16$	$\geq 1/64$
A	181	5 months	106	14
B	43	10 months	22	1
C	7	14 months	7	3
D	12	22 months	6	1
E	16	36 months	12	4

Various measures were used in an effort to control the spread of disease. Herd owners were alerted to the dangers of introducing virus through carrier stock. This resulted in the widespread application of the serum neutralisation test by prospective purchasers of stock. Pigs with positive titres were rejected.

In herds where clinical disease occurred zoosanitary measures were introduced which attempted to confine disease to the initially infected sections. In many instances it soon became apparent that these measures only delayed the spread of

virus within the herd.   Therefore, once disease was confirmed
many producers decided to disseminate virus within the herd as
quickly as possible.   In some herds, as Aujeszky's disease antiserum was not available commercially, serum was harvested from
infected pigs at slaughter.   This was given to piglets at birth
and often produced beneficial results.

However, although many of these control procedures were
useful they failed to halt the advance of Aujeszky's disease,
especially in the larger units.   Therefore, by the late 1970s,
a demand for vaccine was made by the industry.

REFERENCES

Gordon, W.A.M. and Luke, D., 1955.   An outbreak of Aujeszky's disease in
    swine with heavy mortality in piglets, illness in sows, and deaths
    in utero. Vet. Rec. 67, 591-597.
Lamont, H.G., 1946.   Observations on Aujeszky's disease in Northern Ireland.
    Vet. Rec. 58, 621-625.
Lamont, H.G. and Shanks, P.L., 1939.   An outbreak of Aujeszky's disease
    amongst pigs. Vet. Rec. 51, 1407-1408.
McErlean, B.A., 1960.   An outbreak of Aujeszky's disease in piglets.   Irish
    Vet. J. 14, 160-161.
McFerran, J.B. and Dow, C., 1964.   The excretion of Aujeszky's disease
    virus by experimentally-infected pigs.   Res. Vet. Sci. 5, 405-410.
McFerran, J.B., Dow, C. and Hilderbrand, W.R.P., 1966. Aujeszky's disease
    virus. Vet. Rec. 78, 700.
Rosenbaum, M.J., Sullivan, E.J. and Edwards, E.A., 1972. Animal Tissue
    Culture, 1st edition Butterworth's (London) pp 63-67.

AUJESZKY'S DISEASE : CURRENT SITUATION IN BELGIUM

M. Pensaert, L. Maes and K. Andries

Laboratory of Virology, Faculty of Veterinary Medicine,
State University Ghent, Casinoplein 24, B-9000 Ghent,
Belgium.

ABSTRACT

The evolution and current situation of Aujeszky's disease (AD) in Belgium is described. A severe epizootic infection, with a virus strain of high virulence, occurred in 1974 – 76, particularly on breeding farms. A vaccination programme using an inactivated vaccine largely controlled these sudden outbreaks on breeding farms. However, fattening farms then became more and more affected. Thirty-five fattening farms with an outbreak of acute respiratory disorders were examined during the winter period of 1979 – 80. Aujeszky's disease virus, either alone or in combination with swine influenza virus, was found to be associated with 19 of these farms. These outbreaks mainly occurred during the autumn and early winter months.

INTRODUCTION

The evolution of Aujeszky's disease (AD) in Belgium during recent years has not differed very much from that in several other Western European Countries. Although AD virus (ADV) has been known to be present among the Belgian swine population for many years (Van Wassenhove, 1955; Thoonen et al., 1956; Leunen et al., 1975), disease outbreaks were rare and their economic importance was practically nonexistent until the mid seventies. This situation has changed for the worse since 1974 – 75 (Pensaert et al., 1977). Owing to reasons or events still unknown at the present, a virus strain of increased virulence has appeared. This virus strain, serologically identical to the previous one, has manifested itself in at least three different ways:

1. A markedly increased invasiveness within the swine population leading to a sudden increase in the number of outbreaks. A severe epizootic outbreak of AD was first observed in Belgium in 1974 – 76, particularly in regions with a dense swine population.

2. The clinical disease became much more severe due to the fact that the virus-animal interaction is characterised by several tissue tropisms in swine of different ages.

G. Wittmann, S.A. Hall (eds), Aujeszky's Disease. ISBN-13:978-94-009-7555-2

252

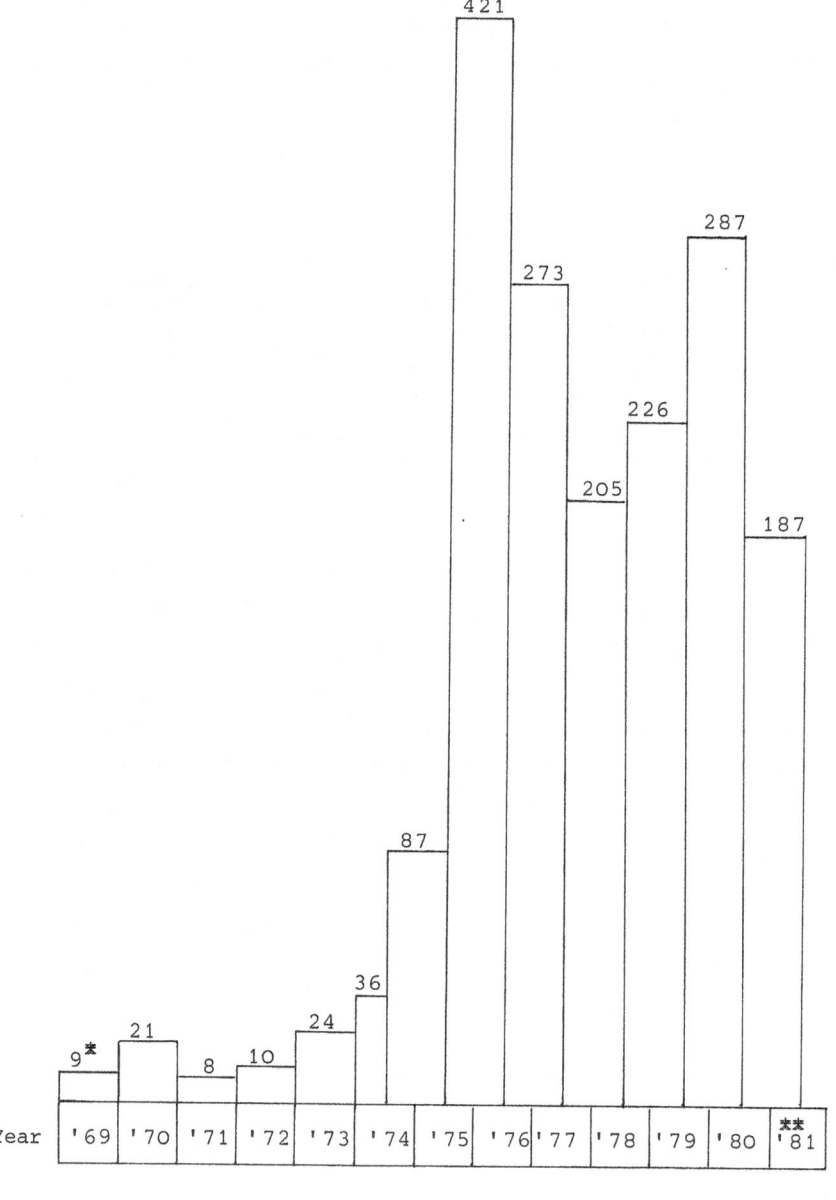

Year | '69 | '70 | '71 | '72 | '73 | '74 | '75 | '76 | '77 | '78 | '79 | '80 | '81

* : Number of diagnosed outbreaks
** : Till April 1981

Fig. 1. Outbreaks of Aujeszky's disease in swine in Belgium.

3. A markedly increased disease incidence upon natural exposure in animal species other than swine.

NUMBER OF OUTBREAKS

The change in the number of outbreaks of AD in swine as recorded in Belgium is presented in Figure 1. It should be pointed out that AD is not a notifiable disease in Belgium. The numbers of outbreaks given in Figure 1 are derived from specific diagnoses made in several diagnostic laboratories on material voluntarily brought in. They do not represent the exact number of outbreaks. Many outbreaks of the disease, particularly in fattening swine, are not known to us. It can be observed that, starting in 1974 - 75, an important epizootic spread of the disease has occurred. In October 1976, a vaccination programme was started on breeding farms (Geskyvac[R] - R. Bellon - inactivated vaccine) (Delagneau et al., 1975). Through this vaccination programme, AD outbreaks have been largely controlled on breeding farms but fattening swine have become more and more affected. AD has, therefore, in recent years become an important problem in fattening swine.

Disease outbreaks are mainly observed during the winter months as shown in Figure 2. For this reason, the numbers presented in Figure 1 have been calculated from July until June of the following calendar year.

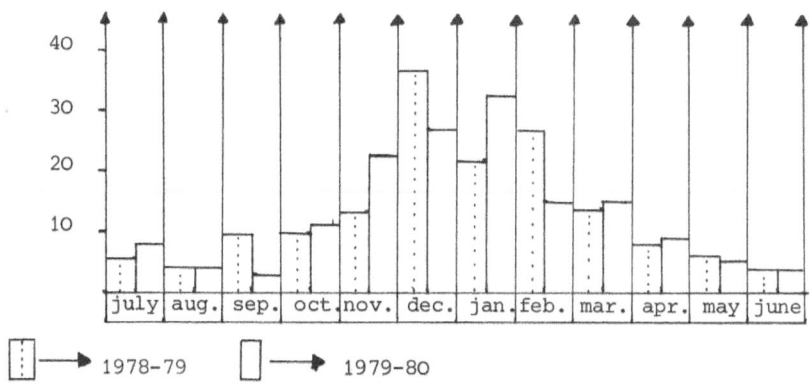

Fig. 2. Monthly distribution of outbreaks of AD (West Flanders).

CLINICAL DISEASE

The animal-virus interaction in swine is characterised by the existence of tropisms for various organs or tissues. Whereas in earlier disease outbreaks in Belgium only piglets became sick, swine of all ages may become infected with the present virus strain of increased virulence. Clinical signs are now characterised mainly by central nervous disorders and death in piglets, by fever, anorexia and abortion in sows and by fever, anorexia, respiratory disorders and weight losses in fattening swine.

A diagnostic study was carried out in our laboratory in order to find out how often ADV is involved in outbreaks of acute respiratory disease on fattening and on breeding swine farms.

Fattening farms

Acute outbreaks of respiratory disease with high morbidity often occur in fattening farms particularly during the winter months. In order to determine the role of ADV in these outbreaks, virological and serological examinations were carried out on 35 farms on which such an outbreak occurred during the winter period of 1979 - 80. Examination was not only directed towards ADV but also towards swine influenza virus, a virus which was shown to be prevalent in Belgium since 1979 (Vandeputte et al., 1980; Pensaert et al., 1981). The results of this study are presented in Table 1.

TABLE 1

VIROLOGICAL EXAMINATION OF ACUTE RESPIRATORY DISEASE ON FATTENING FARMS

Method	Number of farms	Positive for			Negative for
		AD*	Infl.*	AD + infl.	AD and infl.
Virus isolation	26	11	3	5	7
Serology	9	1	4	2	2
Total	35	12	7	7	9

* AD: Aujeszky's disease
* Infl.: Swine influenza (Hsw N1)

It was concluded from these results that the 2 viruses examined were involved in 75% of the respiratory outbreaks. The discovery that these viruses play such an important and causal role is probably due to the fact that only acute outbreaks were selected for this study. When only these virus-induced outbreaks are taken into account, it can be seen that ADV was associated with 75% and swine influenza virus with 54%. In about one quarter of the virus-induced outbreaks (27%), both viruses appeared to be involved at the same time.

Although a clinical differentiation between an AD outbreak and influenza in fattening swine is very difficult to make, some tendencies could be discerned. ADV spread somewhat more slowly throughout the animal population on the farm than influenza virus, its effect was more severe because of the high fever and anorexia and it resulted in marked weight losses. Influenza, on the other hand, had a more explosive character, it disappeared from the farm within 2 to 3 weeks and was of less economic importance. Mortality rates, however, were very variable with both viruses and ranged from 0 to 3%.

It has come to our attention that the majority of typical clinical AD outbreaks in fattening swine occur during the autumn or early winter months. In order to try to find an explanation for this feature, an attempt was made to follow the course of the infection on 5 farms. The total number of animals on these farms varied from 700 to 7 200. On each farm, the animals were housed in different and separate units (300 to 700 animals per unit) which were filled according to the 'all in all out' system. In this study, consecutive groups of weaned pigs, brought in during and after the outbreak, were followed at regular time intervals throughout the fattening period for ADV infection using the skin hypersensitivity test (Vandeputte et al., 1980) or serological examinations.

It was observed that pigs introduced within 2 months after AD had been diagnosed still became systematically infected after arrival. They all built up active immunity which lasted at least until slaughter age, 3 - 4 months later. The high population immunity probably protected these farms from further clinical outbreaks during the winter. However, animals

introduced 3 to 4 months and later after the initial outbreak
had occurred remained negative until slaughter age. The ADV
apparently had then disappeared from the farms. During subsequent months, the population immunity also gradually disappeared. However, the risk of reinfection had already become
very low at that time because the peak season for ADV had
passed during the late spring and summer. No infections occurred during the summer but all the farms became reinfected during
the following autumn or early winter months. At that time, the
virus entered, presumably from outside, into completely susceptible swine populations and this resulted in typical clinical
outbreaks.

Breeding farms

The AD situation on breeding farms has changed in recent
years as a consequence of vaccination. In 1974 and 1975 the
disease occurred as sudden epizootic outbreaks with high morbidity and mortality rates. In recent years, the disease has
become more enzootic. Vaccination of sows using the inactivated vaccine mentioned above (Geskyvac) not only protects the
sows themselves against abortion through active immunity but
also provides efficient protection for the piglets against
central nervous disorders through maternal immunity (Andries
et al., 1976; Andries et al., 1978).

Typical outbreaks of AD on Belgian breeding farms still
occur on farms which have not performed vaccination. An important number of outbreaks also occur on breeding farms on which
the prescribed vaccination schedule has not been followed. In
those cases, central nervous disorders are observed only in
litters from unvaccinated gilts and disease may also be seen in
a few scattered sows. However, if regular vaccination of the
sows is performed, losses from AD in a breeding farm can be
prevented very efficiently.

ADV does not seem to be involved in outbreaks of acute
respiratory disease on breeding farms. A diagnostic study
similar to the one described on the fattening farms was carried
out on 15 breeding farms. The results are presented in Table 2.
All the farms had been vaccinated against ADV.

TABLE 2

VIROLOGICAL EXAMINATION OF ACUTE RESPIRATORY DISEASE ON BREEDING FARMS

Method	Number of farms	Positive for			Negative for
		AD*	Infl.*	AD + Infl.	AD and Infl.
Virus isolation	8	O	2	O	6
Serology	7	O	6	O	1
Total	15	O	8	O	7

* AD: Aujeszky's disease
* Infl.: Swine influenza (Hsw N1)

It can be seen from this table that ADV was never involved, but that influenza virus was a regular cause of the respiratory symptoms. The fact that vaccination was performed on these breeding farms probably did not play a determining role since vaccination of swine with the inactivated vaccine mentioned above does not protect the animals against respiratory infection and disease with ADV (Pensaert et al., 1981).

OTHER ANIMAL SPECIES AFFECTED

Another indication of the increased virulence of the present ADV strain is the number of cases of the disease in animal species such as dogs, cats, cattle and sheep living in direct or indirect contact with infected swine or eating abattoir offal containing virus from swine. Disease in these species has now become a regular feature. During the last 6 years, a specific virological diagnosis has been made in Belgium in 39 cats, 43 dogs and 34 cattle. Although those figures are not by any means representative of the real number of cases, they are at least an indication that the enzootic disease situation in swine means a constant threat for animal species other than swine. AD is, in our experience, always fatal once the infection has started in those animal species.

Vaccination of dogs and cattle using the inactivated vaccine Geskyvac does not result in efficient protection when an intranasal challenge with the virulent virus is given (Pensaert et al., 1980; Biront et al., 1981). It is known that

258

most attenuated vaccines, even if sufficiently harmless to
swine, are still too pathogenic and too dangerous to be applied
to other animal species. Therefore, there are as yet no effective measures for protecting species other than swine.

ACKNOWLEDGEMENTS

We thank Doctors Biront, Leunen, Castryck, De Roose,
Robijns and Segers for contributing the number of outbreaks
diagnosed in their respective laboratories.

The financial support of the Institute for Encouragement
of Scientific Research in Industry and Agriculture (IWONL)
Brussels is gratefully acknowledged.

REFERENCES

Andries, K., Pensaert, M.B., Van Lierde, H., Leunen, J., Castryck, F. and
    De Roose, P., 1976. Vaccinatieproeven met een levende en een
    geïnaktiveerde entstof tegen de ziekte van Aujeszky. Vl. Diergen.
    Tijdschr. 11, 340.
Andries, K., Pensaert, M.B. and Vandeputte, J., 1978. Effect of experimental
    infection with pseudorabies (Aujeszky's disease) virus on pigs with
    maternal immunity from vaccinated sows. Am. J. Vet. Res. 39, 1282-
Biront, P., Vandeputte, J., Pensaert, M.B. and Leunen, J., 1981. Vaccination
    of cattle against Aujeszky's Disease Virus with homologous (Herpes
    suis) and heterologous virus (Herpes bovis 1) - Accepted for public-
    ation in Am. J. Vet. Res. 1981.
Delagneau, J.T., Toma, B., Vannier, P. et al., 1975. Immunisation contre la
    maladie d'Aujeszky à l'aide d'un vaccin Rec. Med. Vet. 151, 567-
Leunen, J., De Meurichy, W. and Pensaert, M., 1975. La maladie d'Aujeszky
    en Belgique, Bull. Off. Int. Epiz. XLIII° session - rapport 207.
Pensaert, M., Castryck, F., Leunen, J. and Vandeputte, J., 1977. Recente
    evolutie en huidige situatie van de ziekte van Aujeszky bij het
    varken in België. Vl. Diergen. Tijdschr. 46, 444-451.
Pensaert, M.B., Commeyne, S. and Andries, K., 1980. Vaccination of Dogs
    against Pseudorabies (Aujeszky's disease) using an inactivated-virus
    vaccine. Am. J. Vet. Res. 41, 12 2016-2019.
Pensaert, M., Ottis, K., Vandeputte, J., Kaplan, M.M. and Bachmann, P.A.,
    1981. Evidence for the natural transmission of influenza A virus
    from wild ducks to swine and its potential importance for men.
    Accepted for publication in W.H.O. Bulletin 1981 - 59(1) 75-78.
Pensaert, M.B., Vandeputte, J. and Andries, K., 1981. Oronasal challenge of
    fattening pigs after vaccination with an inactivated pseudorabies
    vaccine. Accepted for publication in Res. Vet. Sci. 1981.
Thoonen, J., Devos, A., and Hoorens, J., 1956. Ziekte van Aujeszky bij biggen.
    Vl. Diergen. Tijdschr. 3, 68-83.
Vandeputte, J., Pensaert, M. and Castryck, F., 1980. Serologische diagnose
    en onderzoek naar verspreiding van het varkensinfluenzavirus in
    België. Vl. Diergen. Tijdschr. 49, 1-7.
Vandeputte, J. and Pensaert, M.B., 1980. Skin test as herd diagnosis for
    Aujeszky's disease (Pseudorabies) in swine. Vet. Quat. 2, 75-81.
Van Wassenhove, A., 1955. Pseudolyssa in België. Vl. Diergen. Tijdschr.
    2, 35-38.

THE OCCURRENCE AND CONTROL OF AUJESZKY'S DISEASE IN THE FEDERAL REPUBLIC OF GERMANY

H. Pittler

Bundesministerium für Ernährung, Landwirschaft und Forsten, 5300 Bonn, Federal Republic of Germany.

ABSTRACT

The growing problems with Aujeszky's disease (AD) have led the Federal Ministry of Food, Agriculture and Forestry to introduce statutory protection measures. A special regulation for control of AD has been in force since May 8th, 1980. The main aims of state control measures are:
1. The precise registration of all cases of the epizootic disease.
2. The eradication of the disease in infected stock.
3. The protection of stocks and regions free from infection.
4. The limitation of economic losses.

INTRODUCTION

Aujeszky's Disease (AD) has been known for quite a long time but it is only recently, over the past five to six years, that the disease has become of increasing economic and scientific interest in the Federal Republic of Germany.

OCCURRENCE

Figure 1 shows the number of notifications received by the Länder authorites under the regulation of 29 April, 1970 on the reporting of epizootic diseases. The curve shows the rising prevalence of the disease in pigs from 1976/77 and the very steep rise since 1977/78. This trend is also reflected in the figures for cattle as well as for dogs, cats and other animals.

Figure 2 shows the figures for some Federal Länder where the disease has become more or less important. It can be seen that the prevalence of the disease is particularly high in the Federal Länder of Lower Saxony and Nordrhein Westfalen.

The growing problems in general practice, and above all the rising economic importance of the disease in the regions mainly affected, led the Federal Ministry of Food, Agriculture and Forestry to introduce statutory protection measures. A special regulation for control of AD has been in force since 8th May, 1980.

G. Wittmann, S.A. Hall (eds), Aujeszky's Disease. ISBN-13:978-94-009-7555-2

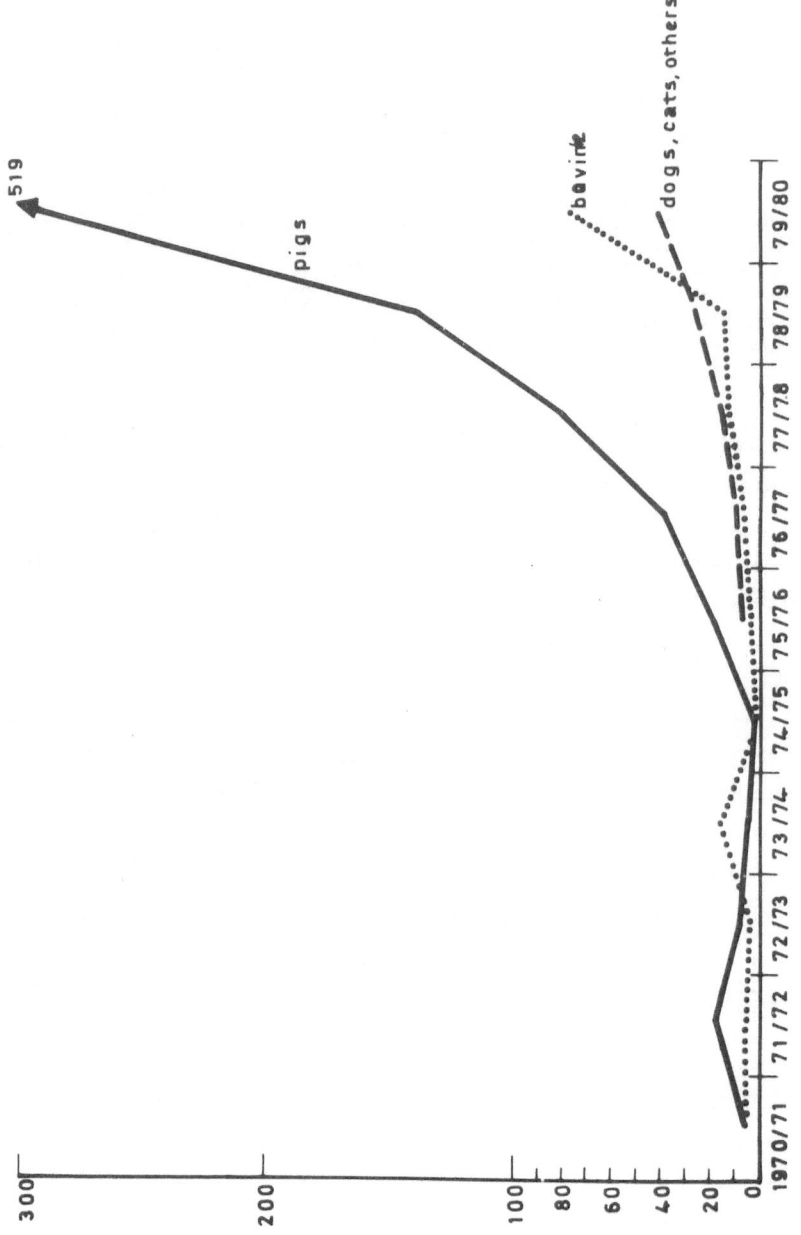

Fig. 1. Aujeszky's Disease, cases after the order from 29.4.1970 - Federal Republic of Germany - (till March 1980).

261

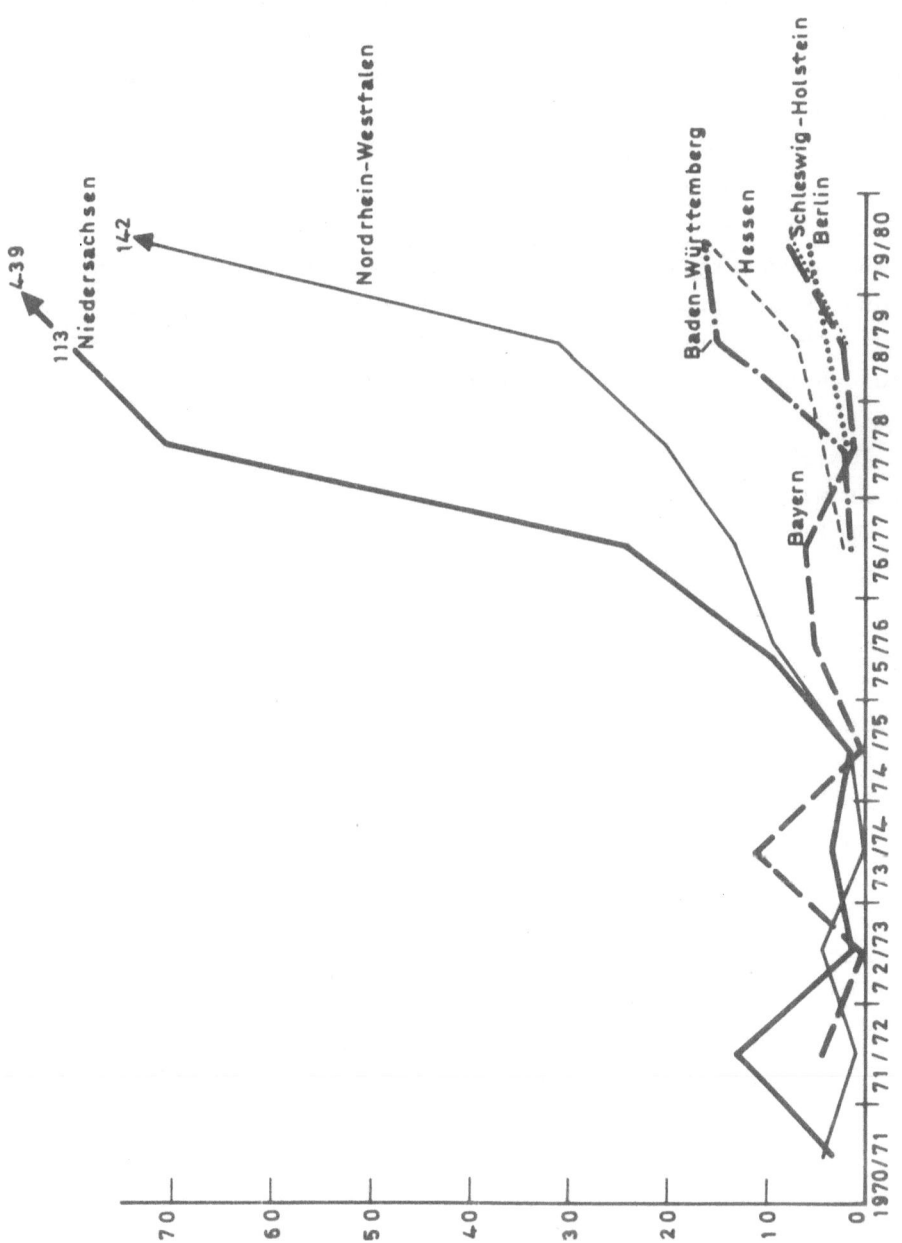

Fig. 2. Aujeszky's Disease, cases after the order from 29.4.1970, Federal Länder (till March 1980).

Figure 3 shows the number of cases of AD (number of farmsteads) that were reported after the establishment of state control measures in May 1980. The areas mainly affected were the Federal Länder of Lower Saxony and Nordrhein Westfalen as can be clearly seen in both Figures 3 and 2. In Lower Saxony a downward trend becomes apparent.

The importance of the disease in pigs is that on farms with pig breeding and pig production the total stock of suckling pigs may die, thus causing considerable economic losses. Losses are also caused by the death of single adult animals, by abortion and by prolonging the fattening period for fattening stocks. There can also be considerable losses in herds of cattle due to the disease causing deaths.

STATE CONTROL

As already mentioned, the regulation for AD came into force on 8th May, 1980. By this order AD became a notifiable disease that must be controlled.

The main aims of state control of AD are:
1. The precise registration of all cases of the epizootic disease.
2. The eradication of the disease in the infected stock.
3. The protection of the stocks and regions free from infection.
4. The limitation of economic losses.

The methods of state control are:
1. Quarantine
2. Disinfection
3. Vaccination
4. Slaughter of animals
5. Disposal or heat treatment of the meat of infected animals.

When deciding on the measures to eradicate or control AD within a herd it is necessary to consider each case individually according to the species, type and size of herd. For pigs the options are:
- to kill all pigs in the herd; this is only applied in the case of smaller herds and extensive infection.

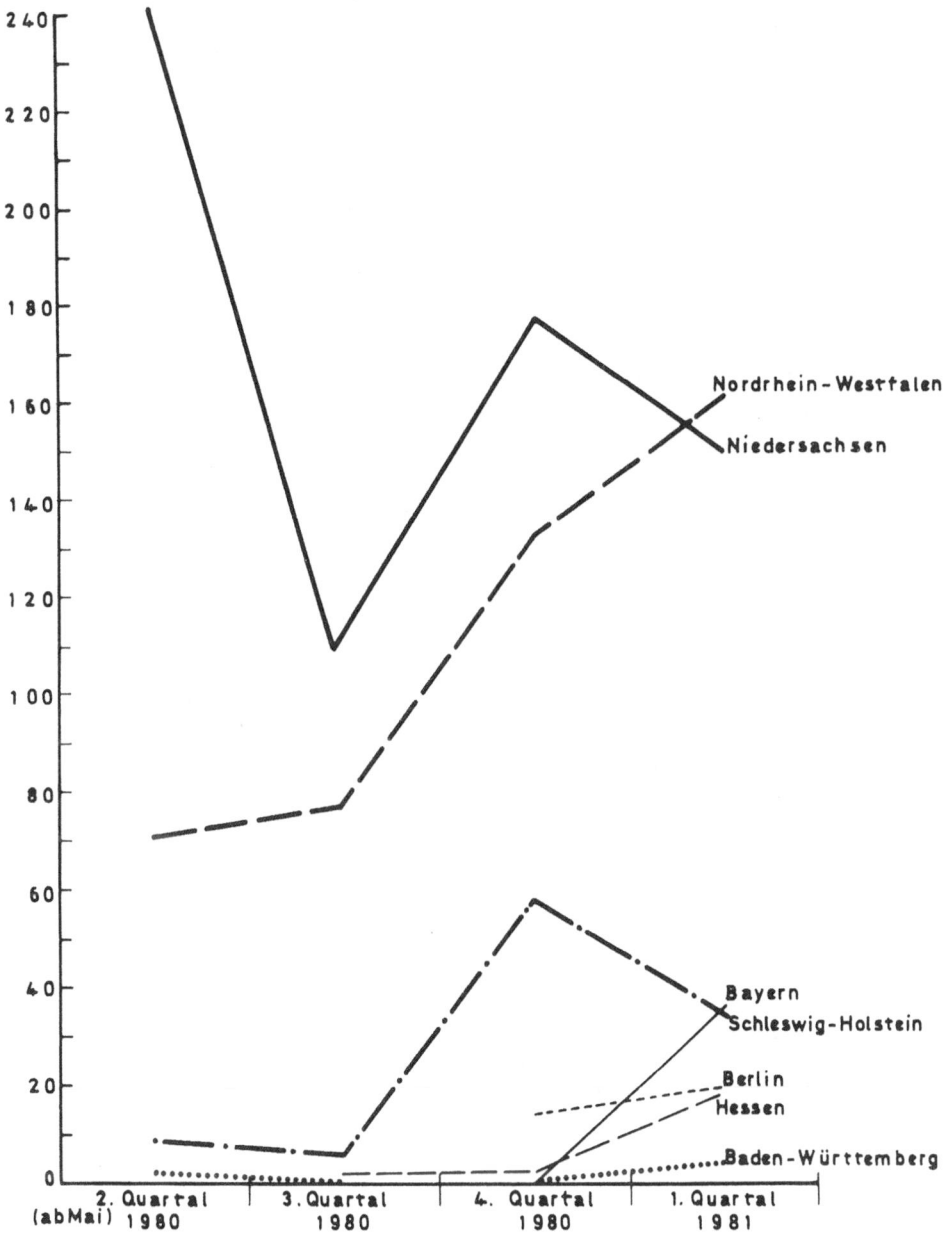

Fig. 3.   Aujeszky's Disease, reported cases after the establishment of order
          from 30.4.1980.

- To kill only the infected or suspect pigs including any of their piglets that are two weeks old or younger, and to examine the remaining pigs serologically twice at an interval of four weeks (if they are older than 3 months); the test must have a negative result.
- To kill all infected and suspect pigs and to vaccinate all remaining animals against AD; in the case of vaccination further infections must not occur in the herd within 35 days and random serologic tests with a negative result must be carried out in piglets born later.

In species other than pigs, infected animals or those suspected of being infected will normally be culled and control measures based on serological tests will be carried out on the remaining animals.

Protection of stocks free from disease

As a precautionary measure it is recommended that owners should have a serological check test done on all breeding stock before being added to the herd (particularly valuable herds).

In herds at high risk from the disease protection may be given by active immunisation but, because of the possible danger of spreading the virus by incubation in vaccinated pigs, the order bans the uncontrolled use of vaccines. Live vaccines are forbidden but the responsible authority may permit the use of inactivated vaccine.

Owners should clearly recognise the necessity for protecting herds that are free from infection and this should be encouraged by making available comprehensive information about the dangers of the disease and its economic impacts.

Import regulations

We have to differentiate between imports of live animals from EC member countries and from third countries. Up to now there have been no regulations regarding AD on intra-Community trade in cattle and pigs and it does not yet appear on the list of notifiable diseases in the so-called regulation on live animals. For some time the Federal Republic of Germany has

made efforts to close this gap in intra-Community trade; it
might be possible to do so by amending directive 64/432, the
so-called live animal directive. We hope that the discussions
from this meeting will be helpful in future work on that topic
in Brussels.

EXPERIMENTAL AUJESZKY'S DISEASE VIRUS INFECTION IN WILD SWINE

F. Tozzini

Istituto di Malattie Infettive,
Facoltà Veterinaria, 56100 Pisa, Italy.

ABSTRACT

Experimental infection with Aujeszky's disease virus was carried out by the oral route in four young wild swine. No symptoms were observed but the virus was shed in the oral discharge with subsequent infection of the control animals. The virus was reisolated from the tonsil, but not from lung or brain; subsequently the throat swabs became negative also. Multiplication of the virus in the host was confirmed by the raising of the specific neutralising antibodies.

INTRODUCTION

The presence of a large number of wild swine in Italy and increased breeding and crossing with domesticated swine led us to consider their susceptibility to Aujeszky's disease virus (ADV). In the past we had occasion to suspect these animals as transmitters of Aujeszky's disease (AD) when dogs died from confirmed AD after being bitten by wild boars during hunting.

The only information we could find on this subject in the literature dates from 1913; it concerns a case of AD occurring naturally in wild swine (Ratz, St. Von, 1913).

We have therefore conducted research on experimental transmission in young wild swine using a virulent ADV strain. The results will be reported in detail in a paper now in press (Tozzini et al., 1981); on the occasion of this meeting we intend to present some of the information.

MATERIALS AND METHODS

Six 16 week old wild swine were used. Four were infected by the oral route with different amounts of the virus (from 10^5 to $10^{6.3}$ TCID$_{50}$). The animals were observed daily for signs of the disease. At intervals the swine were captured; throat, nasal and conjunctival swabs and blood samples were collected until slaughter when the organs were sent to the laboratory for the virological procedures. PK15 cell cultures were used for isolation of the virus and the serum-neutralisation test.

G. Wittmann, S.A. Hall (eds), Aujeszky's Disease. ISBN-13:978-94-009-7555-2

RESULTS

No signs or symptoms of AD developed in the six animals during the course of the experiment - that is 10 to 42 days post infection. In each animal infected by the oral route, the virus was recovered from throat swabs. In one subject it appeared also in the nasal swab and in another in the conjunctival swab. The shedding of virus lasted 5 - 12 days and caused an infection in the control swine living in the same house. Virological tests carried out on organs of the animals slaughtered at various intervals indicated the presence of virus in the tonsils of only three animals. In one of these pigs the throat swab was also positive but in the other two the throat swab had been negative for 3 days and 9 days respectively prior to slaughter. In the animals slaughtered later, the virological procedures carried out on the tonsils were negative indicating that after 15 - 30 days from the end of the oral shedding period, the virus cannot be recovered from the tonsil. Reisolation tests conducted on organs such as lungs, brain and lymphnodes were negative. This was in agreement with the results of the immunofluorescence test that resulted positive only with sections of tonsil from which the virus had been reisolated. The results of the serum neutralisation test showed a progressive increase of specific antibody titres during the course of the experiment in all the wild swine - a further demonstration of virus multiplication in the animal body.

CONCLUSIONS

The results show that the inoculation of virulent ADV into the oral cavity of 16 week old wild swine caused an asymptomatic infection with shedding and transmission of the virus to cohabitant wild swine. The subsequent recovery of virus from the tonsils of the animals after throat swabs had become negative suggests that wild swine may also be carriers, as already indicated for the domestic pig (McFerran and Dow, 1964; 1965). Assuming that the shedding of the virus and its prolonged presence in the tonsils might occur naturally in wild swine, they must be considered a potential danger for domestic swine and dogs in relation to local customs of commerce and hunting. The persistence of the virus in the tonsils or in other tissues could subsequently induce an additional shedding of the virus in relation to stress associated with trapping or transportation by truck, which is the custom in our region.

REFERENCES

McFerran, J.B. and Dow, C., 1964. The excretion of Aujeszky's disease
    virus by experimentally infected pigs. Res. Vet. Scien. 5, 405.
McFerran, J.B. and Dow, C., 1965. The distribution of the virus of
    Aujeszky's disease in experimentally infected swine. Amer. Jour.
    Vet. Res. 26, 112.
Ratz, St. Von., 1913. in Lautie, R., 1969. Les maladies à virus. La mala-
    die d'Aujeszky. Expansion Scient. Franc.
Tozzini, F., Poli, A. and Della Croce, G., 1981. In press.

FIELD EXPERIENCE WITH AUJESZKY'S DISEASE
IN THE UNITED KINGDOM

E.N. Wood

Veterinary Investigation Centre,
Norwich, NR6 6ST, UK.

ABSTRACT

The incidence of Aujeszky's disease (AD) in Britain and the clinical signs of disease in East Anglian pig herds are described. Serious respiratory and reproductive symptoms are not a common feature of AD in this region.

Lesions visible to the naked eye and having the histological characteristics of AD were found in the liver, tonsil, gut or skin in 15/25 incidents investigated.

Compared to the numbers reported in other EC countries, there have been very few cases of Aujeszky's disease (AD) in pig herds in Britain. The number of new outbreaks in any one year has never exceeded 34. This year (1981) only 5 had been recorded by the end of May. At present, there are probably no more than 100 infected herds in Britain. Most are in East Anglia, which is an area of high pig density.

The clinical picture seen in outbreaks of AD in East Anglia varies greatly. Affected fattening herds often suffer little or no economic loss. In these herds mortality has not exceeded 1%, that is, it has been no more than that expected in normal unaffected herds. Food conversion has been within 0.1 of unaffected contemporaries. This is in contrast to hearsay reports from some other countries of significant losses in fattening units. Breeding herds often exhibit the expected characteristic signs. Sows show anorexia and depression, usually lasting for four days, while young piglets, three weeks of age or less, shake, shiver, make convulsive movements and die. However, the reproductive failure which is frequently referred to in the literature has rarely occurred. Most reports of poor reproductive performance have been based on assessments made by the farmer himself. Reports of this kind are obviously open to criticism. Ministry of Agriculture officers at our headquarters at Tolworth estimate that each outbreak of AD is accompanied by

only 2 cases of abortion per 100 sows. This is little more
than the normal incidence given by Pepper et al. (1977). It
is certainly less than 2.5%, the level at which these authors
recommend that action should be taken. Reproductive disorders
play only a small role in outbreaks of AD in East Anglia and
many herds suffer no adverse effects from poor breeding performance even when, in other respects, they experience an outbreak that is typical of this disease. Only rarely have significant losses been due to reproductive failure, and rarely
has this aspect been investigated fully and laboratory confirmation obtained.

Similarly, there is little evidence that respiratory
disease is an important manifestation of AD: farmers with
infected herds in East Anglia seldom describe sneezing or
coughing as part of the problem.

Some medium-sized herds (100 sows or more) infected with
AD virus have shown few of the characteristic clinical signs
(anorexia in sows and nervous symptoms in young piglets) but
only a temporary increase in the incidence and severity of
neonatal diarrhoea.

Why does the severity of symptoms vary so much on neighbouring units when circumstantial evidence suggests that
infection has spread from one to the other? It has been
suggested that the stage of pregnancy of sows at the time of
initial infection influences the severity of clinical signs.
I cannot except this because most East Anglian herds are large
enough to contain sows at all stages of pregnancy at all times.

There are many references in the literature to histopathological changes but very few references in the English
language to lesions visible to the naked eye. An exception is
the very good description by Finazzi and Mandelli of Italy
(1976).

My own experience has been that macroscopic lesions were
found in 15 of 25 recent outbreaks from which piglets (between
2 and 8 in number) were examined *post mortem*. The affected piglets showed many small cream foci, 1 - 2 mm in diameter, on
the surface and in the substance of the liver. Similar lesions
occurred in the spleen. Lesions as small as this could easily

be missed in the field but should be clearly visible in a
careful *post mortem* examination carried out in a laboratory.
They were found in pigs of 1 - 3 weeks of age. When these
lesions were seen, further examination of the piglets - or of
other piglets in the same litter - always resulted in confirmation of AD by virus isolation and/or serology. In many cases
histopathological examination of lesions showed the presence of
intranuclear inclusion bodies, leaving little if any doubt that
they were caused by AD virus. The lesions are distinct foci of
coagulative necrosis, sometimes confluent and often subcapsular.
They contain some cellular detritus and the edge of the lesion
often shows cellular infiltration. Acidophilic intranuclear
inclusion bodies with vascular degeneration and disintegration
occur, particularly in the larger lesions. The histopathology
is described in more detail in the Italian paper referred to
above.

In 3 of the 15 incidents, lesions occurred in the tonsils,
some of which were covered by a diphtheritic membrane. Histologically, inclusions were found in the epithelial cells lining
the crypts. There was also polymorphonuclear cell infiltration
at the edge of the lesions.

Lesions were rarely seen in the gut. When present, they
occurred in the jejunum and appeared as small areas of necrosis
2 mm in diameter. Histopathology showed focal necrotic lesions
in the muscle coats. Acidophilic intranuclear inclusions were
present, supporting the suggestion that the lesions were caused
by AD virus.

Baskerville et al. (1973) reported that skin lesions were
present in 2 of 154 outbreaks that they had studied. They also
stated that some other workers considered that skin lesions
were not a feature of AD in the pig.

In one East Anglian incident 3 of a litter of 6 six-day-
old piglets were found with pruritis and skin lesions. The
farmer described the lesions as 'spots or blisters', but on
examination a day later no evidence of vesiculation was present.
Small areas of apparent necrosis were found on the epithelial
surfaces of the mouth and snout and on the skin of the head.
Histological examination showed focal coagulative necrosis

involving the epidermis and hair follicles. In some areas
the necrosis extended into the dermis. Intranuclear inclusion
bodies were found and AD virus was isolated from samples of
skin.

In 15 out of 25 recent outbreaks lesions of coagulative
necrosis were visible to the naked eye at *post mortem*. When
these lesions are observed AD should be suspected even if the
usual clinical signs are absent. In my opinion, these macroscopic lesions have not been given the emphasis they deserve.

REFERENCES

Baskerville, A., McFerran, J.B. and Dow, C., 1973. Aujeszky's Disease in
      Pigs. Vet. Bull., 43, 465-480.
Finazzi, M. and Mandelli, G., 1976. The gross and histological findings in
      the liver of pigs with Aujeszky's disease. Folia vet latina, 6, 368-
      376.
Pepper, T.A., Boyd, H.W. and Rosenberg, P., 1977. Breeding record analysis
      in pig herds and its veterinary applications - 1: Development of a
      program to monitor reproduce efficiency and weaner production. Vet.
      Rec., 101, 177-180.

GENERAL DISCUSSION

J.B. McFerran   (UK)   I was very impressed by Dr. Bitsch's work
this morning.   I find it very interesting that we apparently do
not have many syncytia-forming strains of virus and we are not
seeing lateral spread.   We do have virulent strains so I would
like to look at these strains in more detail.   Could Dr. Bitsch
tell us the exact technique he uses?   Do you stain cover slips?
Do you count the number of syncytia, if so, how many per field
constitute a syncytia-forming strain, etc. ?

V. Bitsch   (Denmark)   We have tested several cells for their
ability to support the formation of syncytia and we found the
cells that most regularly produced or reproduced results were
primary pig kidney cell cultures.

   We do not stain the cultures, we just observe for presence
of syncytia and the difference between the results from non
syncytia strains and syncytia-forming strains is very pronounced.
In a few cases it was difficult to conclude whether it was a
syncytia-forming strain or not and at first we called these
intermediate strains but then we decided that there was no real
reason to have a third group and we have called these doubtful
cases non-syncytia-forming strains.

   There will be differences if you test other cell cultures
because even if one preparation of certain cells gives excellent
results, you may have difficulties when you perform another test
on the basis of the same cells.   PK15 cells, for example, vary
from one preparation of the cells to another.   However, primary
pig kidney cells have worked excellently so far.

Rosalind Gaskell   (UK)   Have you tried plaquing them?   Is there
any difference in plaque size between the two types?

V. Bitsch   No, I haven't.

B. Liess   (Federal Republic of Germany)   Dr. Bitsch, you are not
afraid of any contamination in the primary pig kidney culture
by other viruses?   Adenovirus, for example, which is widespread?

V. Bitsch   You might expect such things in cell lines as well.
The only thing that we have found is that it works when you use
primary pig kidney cells.

<u>B. Liess</u> Would you not expect the risk in a cell line to be much less than in a primary culture?

<u>V. Bitsch</u> Well, we have seen no difference from one estimation of a series of isolates to another, from one evaluation of a series of isolates to another, or another evaluation of the same series of isolates. So I do not fear any interference from viruses being present in the cells that are used for the evaluation.

<u>M. Pensaert</u> (Belgium) Dr, Bitsch, is the quantity of virus inoculated important? We have the feeling that if you inoculate let's say 10^6, 10^7, then most of those strains are syncytia-forming. Is this an important factor?

<u>V. Bitsch</u> Not as far as we have seen. In a routine evaluation we inoculate high doses of virus into the cells. We have also tried low doses of virus and we have seen no differences that could be attributed to the low dose of virus used.

<u>H. Ludwig</u> (Federal Republic of Germany) I think that this syncytia formation will be a very important marker. I think that Dr. Bitsch has controlled all these strains by neutralisation so it will be ADV and it eliminates the possibility that one has a contaminant. I must confess that I got a strain 15 years ago which I published in an unimportant journal as an Aujeszky virus and now by using the restriction enzyme I have found that it is an adenovirus.

It seemed to me that the rounding-up strains were localised more in the back part of the animal, the other in the front of the animal. If this is so, it reminds me of HSV and IBR-IPV situations where they have some serological differences. Can you sero-diagnose? Can you find differences with your sensitive technique, different 'serotypes'?

<u>V. Bitsch</u> Regarding your first comment, I do not know whether it would be a valuable tool to distinguish between strains of high and low pathogenicity. What we have found refers to the conditions in Denmark. Dr. Toma sent us about 20 strains from France and all these were found to be syncytia-forming strains. Conditions in other countries may well be different from the

conditions that we have.

With regard to the identification of the virus strains, we identify our isolates routinely by a direct immunofluorescence test on infected cells from the cell cultures.

With regard to the fact that we have found that the isolates from cattle with posterior pruritus were in all cases non-syncytia-forming strains, we think that there might be a similar situation in AD as in IBR infection in cattle. Some strains may be exclusively respiratory strains, and these strains are highly pathogenic. Some strains might be genital strains and these strains are of lower pathogenicity, and in Denmark are found predominantly in small herds where the infection has obviously been introduced by boars from boar centres. This might be a similar condition.

J.B. Andersen (Denmark) I totally agree with what Dr. Bitsch has just said, that there are these differences.

H. Ludwig Perhaps by adding trypsin it would be possible to cleave that fusion protein and make it a virulent strain?

V. Bitsch We have not had time to do this.

H. Ludwig Maybe I should make one comment about fusion. I think that in herpes virology it is accepted that we only have fusion from within. Classical fusion does not occur, as in Sendai virus, it comes from active replication. A few years ago, we tested fusion factors and I think it depends very much on the cell as to whether it fuses or not.

F. Castrijk (Belgium) Dr. Bitsch, did you see pruritus in all cases in cattle?

V. Bitsch Not in all cases, but in most. There was one case with an anterior site of virus multiplication with posterior sites of multiplication of the virus, without pruritus. We have had several cases where there has been no pruritus in herds where other animals showed anterior localisation of pruritus. It is not a regular phenomenon, but it does occur in most cases.

J.B. Andersen If there are no further questions on this topic I could ask whether any of you have any comments on these problems of AD; disease control, infection control, control and

eradication programmes, especially in relation to vaccination.
Are there any comments on the more practical approaches to the
control programmes that have been mentioned?

P. Vannier   (France)   I think personally that it would be impossible to eradicate AD except by stamping it out.   certainly
think it is impossible to eradicate it by vaccinatiʋn.   Countries
that are lucky enough to have a low level of infection must
quickly begin to practise a sanitary programme otherwise in
five or ten years they too will have an irreversible situation.

J.B. Andersen   I entirely agree that we cannot eradicate by
vaccination but perhaps it can help in the primary phases of
an infection control programme.   It is our experience in Denmark
that situations can exist where test and slaughter policy can be
used within a herd; in most cases I agree that stamping out and
restocking would be the correct policy.   I therefore believe
that it is important that countries with a low prevalence of AD
should make up their minds now whether to have an eradication
programme or disease control.

J.B. McFerran   I agree that we can either go to direct slaughter
on the farm or else attempt to get the next generation from that
farm free by serological testing.   I think that the feasibility
of this will very much depend on the type of virus concerned.
If you have the virus which is giving lateral spread I doubt
very much whether the second possibility that I mentioned is
practical.   If, however, you have the more traditional strains
of virus, then it is possible.   In fact, we have done this on
large farms and it is relatively easy because of the poor
spreading ability of the virus.   On these farms I feel that
vaccination would also be a great help, especially the live
vaccine which would reduce the amount of virulent virus being
excreted.   I know that many people do not like live vaccine but
I think that if the right live vaccine is chosen and it is used
in a situation where you are going to slaughter off those
animals anyway, then it is the preferable choice.

J.B. Andersen   That is a very fundamental statement that you
are making.   We need some pressure to take the steam out of the

bottle! It is our experience that in some heavily infected areas and with highly pathogenic strains that you must in one way or another try to reduce the virus load. I therefore agree totally with what you said about the different strains. The traditional strains are tending towards self eradication in small herds. It is obvious that in such cases a test and slaughter policy could be used. So it all depends on the specific case - both in regard to the herd and the type of virus concerned. For the highly pathogenic and lateral spreading viruses I agree it is quite difficult.

J.B. McFerran   I would like to come back on another point. Clearly there has been a change in the ability of the virus to spread. This also appears to be associated with changes in the behaviour of the virus in the pig. For instance, Dr. Wood described AD in one part of England and the type of disease that he described is unknown to me. In that area he has obviously got area spread; it is obviously very similar to the types of AD that have been described in other parts of Europe, and was indeed described many years ago from Hungary and Czechoslovakia and more recently from the mid-west of the USA where you are seeing lesions in the viscera and skin and seeing pruritus. The old traditional strains did not behave this way. Can we draw a general conclusion that if you start seeing visceral lesions you are dealing with a strain that has the ability to spread laterally?

J.B. Andersen   I am not an expert in this field but I would guess that it may not be so much a change in the strains as a movement of them.

A. Baskerville   (UK)   What Dr, McFerran has said is quite true, but Dr. Wood, in his paper, was saying that he saw very little disease in fattening pigs, whereas the visceral, kidney and liver lesions such as he described, are certainly associated - in the mid-west of the USA, the Far East and other parts of Europe - with a very virulent virus in fattening pigs, with a very high mortality rate of perhaps over 50%. I find it rather strange that in this area of England we have these occasional visceral lesions with an apparently very low virulence virus, compared with the general world experience.

Sheila Cartwright *(UK)* We isolated the virus on tissue culture from that particular outbreak where the visceral and skin lesions were seen. We put it into various age groups and it caused, what to us, was typical AD with nervous signs in the little pigs but no mortality in the older age group. Even though it was different in the field, in the laboratory it behaved like the majority of strains we have isolated in that part of England.

J.B. McFerran I was careful to differentiate before between 'spreadability' and virulence. We have virulent strains that are capable of killing fattening pigs but we do not have lateral spread and we do not have visceral lesions.

V. Bitsch Even if we now see that more pathogenic strains have been spread in parts of the country, we do not regularly see necrotic lesions in the liver of infected piglets. I think that we have seen this in four or five cases, that is all, and the first case we saw was in 1968. We do not see pruritus in pigs, so the higher pathogenicity that we see in Denmark is not associated with a more pronounced occurrence of pruritus or of visceral lesions.

Rosalind Gaskell We have been discussing the various levels of virulence of the virus and how that behaves. Should we not also consider the differences in the host - genetic strains, the presence of other pathogenic agents, bacteria, other viruses, and differences in husbandry, for accounting for quite a lot of this difference in virulence in the field?

J.B. McFerran No, you can take different strains, for instance, the NIA-1 strain and the NIA-3 strain in the same stock of SPF pigs, and the same dose of virus will give entirely different mortalities.

Rosalind Gaskell Yet we have just heard that Dr. Wood's isolate behaved differently in the field in East Anglia from your experimental pigs. It did not produce skin and visceral lesions. In the field that strain behaved differently from experimental pigs even though you can get a fairly standard response in experimental pigs.

Sheila Cartwright Yes, for that one particular case but this
might possibly have been a case where the pigs were actually
infected *in utero* and displaying different signs. They were
very young, about 6 days old, so there are maybe explanations
for that particular case. It was a very exceptional case for
our country.

K. Dalsgaard *(Denmark)* Was this isolate passaged in cell
culture before it was re-inoculated in your laboratory?

Sheila Cartwright The original first passage on pig kidney
culture was put into the experimentally infected piglets.

H. Ludwig Why are we surprised that we should have different
strains? The genetic make-up of an animal influences the
spread of disease and a highly bred animal might be more susceptible to certain viruses. It is known that there are
different strains in other herpes viruses which preferentially
go to the brain etc., and I think in this case of Dr. Wood that
it might be a strain that has a strong virulence and by spreading into the liver it will certainly kill the animal. I do not
think that this is an immune response, it is a necrotic lesion
by virus replication. A little antigenic change in the make-up
of the virion which is not expressed in the DNA is enough to
change the virulence. We know about this in other viruses that
make re-assortment which we can explain, as in influenza. In
the herpes virus, passage in a certain pig population may change
its virulence.

Rosalind Gaskell Does anyone know the reasons for the increased
susceptibility of the young pig to AD? Is it because of the
macrophage system not being sufficient, or is it a temperature
factor, as it is with other herpes virus infections, such as
the canine herpes virus, which increases the susceptibility of
the young animal to the disease?

H. Ludwig Perhaps I can speculate a little here! It is known
that the young animal will always be more susceptible to a

herpes virus. Babies are killed by HSV-1. If there was a full
capacity of immune response you might get rid of the disease.
So this is one factor, the immune response.

The other factor might be that the virus in the animal
might occupy the place to re-infect.

Sheila Cartwright Has anyone any suspicion that there might be
a foetopathic strain of AD, one that does not manifest itself
in normal clinical signs like nervous disease in little piglets,
but that just goes on causing abortion and reproductive failure?

V. Bitsch Whenever we have isolated the virus from aborted or
stillborn foetuses, we have seen the usual clinical symptoms in
young pigs, but we can say that in these cases the clinical
course of the disease in the herds was more serious than seen
in most herds. I do not think you can have a virus that will
appear only as abortogenic and not causing clinical disease in
pigs.

Sheila Cartwright In the West Country, where the cases of AD
are not so typical as those in the eastern part of England, we
have picked three cases showing a rise in the antibody titre to
ADV at the same time as there is reproductive failure in the
herd. We have followed these herds through and at no time have
there been typical clinical signs of the disease, simply this
period of reproductive failure. In one herd we cleared it up
serologically and immediately the reproductive performance
returned to normal. I just wondered if it was a possibility?

Dr. Brovas (Greece) Dr. Gaskell was asking about the nervous
symptoms in piglets, whether there is an age factor here. I
think there may be a parallel with foot and mouth disease. I
am not talking about foot and mouth disease in the field but
rather under experimental conditions. It is well known to
research workers that unweaned mice, up to the seventh day of
life, are susceptible to foot and mouth virus. It is necessary
to adapt the virus otherwise the mice are pathogenic up to the

7th or 8th day, but no longer. They die with nervous symptoms - paralysis followed by death.

P. Vannier *(France)* I think that the question raised by Dr. Gaskell is very important. There is a lack of knowledge in this area. Such knowledge might clarify the situation about the virulence of the strain. I would like to take the example of TGE. We know more about the pathogenicity of the TGE virus and we know why young piglets are much more sensitive to the action of TGE virus in comparison with adult animals. It is a question of the pH in the stomach, a question of the speed of cell renewal in the gut, and many other factors. I do not think that we know much about this in AD and it would be a help in discovering the different virulence of the strains.

P.W. de Leeuw *(Netherlands)* Going back to the question about the role of macrophages, we have thought about this and we have tried to make growth curves of different virus strains of AD in macrophage cultures of SPF pigs of about one week of age. We have not followed it up lately because we found there is no clear pattern. Some virulent strains grew quite well in macrophage cultures but at the same time we found adapted strains like the Bartha strain that also grew quite well. There was no clear pattern at all.

B. Liess I would still like to know something about the determination of virulence. How can the virulence of the strains be determined?

P.W. de Leeuw We have compared a number of strains, although not as many as we should have. You take seronegative SPF pigs of the same age and weight, challenge these intranasally with a fixed amount of virus in both nostrils and then follow it up. If you take all the pigs the mortality will be low. You then use weight curves and express this in terms of the time it takes them to regain their original weight, or if you take younger pigs you can take the mortality. We have used weight curves.

SUMMARY AND CONCLUSIONS

G. Wittmann, J.B. Andersen, P.W. de Leeuw and B. Toma

In the section 'Properties of Aujeszky's disease virus (ADV)' reports dealt with the analysis of ADV-DNAs of field isolates with partly different biological properties, and of modified live virus vaccine strains by cleavage with restriction endonucleases. It was found that this technique may well prove to be an adequate tool for unambiguous identification of ADV isolates from the field. Based on the DNA patterns field major classes of ADV strains could be constructed. The investigations are only beginning but one hopes that they will he in the future to find connections between DNA and biological properties, especially virulence of the virus strains. Besides, with the aid of DNA analysis it is now possible to check if live vaccine strains retain their genetic stability after subpassages in the host.

Attempts have been made to investigate the major immunogenic proteins and antigens of ADV. Indirect immunoprecipitation tests revealed that up to 10 proteins, ranging in molecular weights between 40 000 and 200 000 daltons were recognised by convalescent sera from pigs. Six of these proteins were glycosylated. In preliminary experiments it was shown that at least one major immunogenic component could be identified as a glycoprotein. These investigations can be of importance for the development of better inactivated vaccines and sub-unit vaccines.

As concerns the biological differentiation of virulent ADV strains and modified live virus vaccines, no genetic marker has been known until now which is absolutely coupled with pig virulence. However, there are attenuated strains a few markers of which differ from those of field strains.

In the section 'Diagnostic procedures' serology was the main topic. Seroneutralisation is until now the reference technique for serological diagnosis and for studying humoral immunity in AD. The sensitivity of the neutralisation test can be largely enhanced by incubation of the serum-virus mixture during 24 hours at $37^{\circ}C$. Thereby a thermoresistant virus strain has to be used or thermal inactivation has to be regarded. A further increase of sensitivity can be achieved by the addition of guinea pig complement.

The enzyme-linked immunosorbent assay (ELISA) is a new test which demands attention for the serological diagnosis of AD. Its advantages (high sensitivity, high specificity, quick performance, partial automatisation and lower price than the neutralisation test) will certainly lead to the replacement of the neutralising test by ELISA for mass screening of sera.

The participants of the seminar accepted a conclusion in which the necessity of standardisation of the results of sero- logical tests on Aujeszky's disease was underlined. However, it was stated that it is quite impossible that all laboratories use the same technique, the same cell strain, the same virus strain and so on. Nevertheless, it is desirable that all laboratories have in common a reference serum for comparing the sensitivity of their tests. First steps have been taken in the meanwhile to implement this suggestion.

Erroneous virological diagnosis of AD as a result of the preceding use of live vaccines can occur. This risk can be reduced when histopathological examinations and immuno- fluorescence are employed, since the degree of the alterations is lower after live vaccination than after infection with virulent virus.

In the section 'Immunity and pathogenesis' it became obvious that in contrast to humoral immunity, which has been investigated very well, the role of IgA, interferon, and cell- mediated immunity (CMI) should not be neglected, since CMI is supposed to be the main factor in recovery from herpes virus infections, whereas humoral immunity is thought to prevent infection. However, it was recently shown, that infection with high amounts of virus is not prevented by antibodies. There- fore, further work should be done to clarify the relationship between IgA in the nasal, tracheal and pharyngeal secretions and IgA, IgM and IgG in the serum on the one hand and the amount of virus necessary to penetrate this antibody barrier on the other hand.

After vaccination with inactivated vaccines it was found that the pigs showed a much more restricted antibody profile in crossed immunoelectrophoresis than infected animals. It was demonstrated that these antibodies were directed mainly against glycoprotein antigens of ADV. These results indicate that the presence of the glycoprotein complex in inactivated vaccines may play a significant role for the protection of vaccinated animals. Further work in this field is necessary, especially with regard to efficacy testing of inactivated AD vaccines.

After intranasal ADV infection of cattle it was demonstrated that the virus multiplies in the naso-pharyngeal region and penetrates from there the central nervous system (CNS) via the neural pathways. The finding that virus was shed by some of the cattle in the nasal excretion with titres up to $10^{3.5}TCD_{50}$ per swab, offers the possibility that ADV infected cattle may be a source of infection for other animals. Since a rather low level of ADV ($10^{4}TCD_{50}$) can be sufficient to infect cattle it seems to be possible that transmission of infection to cattle may occur by air, contaminated food and implements, and by man.

In the section 'Vaccination' results of comparative trials in pigs were presented which suggested that even the best vaccines available, be it attenuated or inactivated, will only reduce the amount of virus shed after natural exposure. Since in the trials challenge was performed two weeks p.v., one may assume that in the field, where longer intervals will occur, the decrease in virus shedding of vaccinated pigs after exposure will become less and less marked. These findings provide further evidence for the by now widely held opinion that vaccination of pigs against AD will not limit the spread of the disease, but will only reduce economic losses. A decrease of economic losses has also been observed by many field workers when vaccination was started immediately after the onset of an outbreak, particularly if a good attenuated vaccine was available. The results obtained with an inactivated vaccine were no less than those obtained with an attenuated vaccine. The rapid development of protection that was observed after

vaccination could not be fully explained, indicating the need
for more fundamental immunological research in the field of AD.

In some regions vaccination of pigs from immunised dams
constitutes a major problem. It was found that an inactivated
vaccine was much less effective in pigs with maternal antibodies than in sero-negative pigs. A second vaccination was
not tried and it might have given better results, but in the
case of fatteners the cost might then become prohibitive. The
problem of interference of maternal antibodies with active
immunisation is not only limited to the use of inactivated vaccines but also occurs when using attenuated vaccines. Although
appreciating the complexity of the problem of interference, it
is undoubtedly important enough, particularly in fatteners, to
warrant further study. One approach may be intranasal instead
of parenteral vaccination with live vaccines. It was reported
that a single intranasal vaccination against AD was even more
effective than two parenteral vaccinations with the same
attenuated strain of virus. With regard to inactivated vaccines
the blockade of active immunisation by passive immunity should
be the subject of further work. The use of more potent adju-
vants, higher antigen doses and proper vaccination schemes may
be promising.

The performance of AD-virus vaccines in the field is
difficult to evaluate and the epizootiological situation should
be taken into account. For instance, under the relatively
favourable disease situation in the Republic of Ireland an
American inactivated vaccine appeared to give promising results.
On the other hand, in Italy it was observed that of a locally
produced inactivated and an attenuated vaccine, the latter was
considerably more effective than the former in controlling the
disease in strongly infected areas.

The issue of inactivated versus attenuated vaccines in
general was not discussed in depth. In the opinion of the
writers such a discussion is difficult to hold in a sensible
manner anyway, as one cannot generalise in this field. Many
vaccines of each type are now available and the information on
each should be carefully studied. Another problem is that data
on their efficacy, obtained under comparable conditions, are

lacking. Finally the epizootiological situation in a particular region will also influence the appraisal of a vaccine. The
question was raised whether, for safety reasons, more emphasis
should be placed on the development of sub-unit vaccines, i.e.
vaccines lacking the viral genome. It was pointed out that
research in this area is under way, but that even if such vaccines will eventually prove to be effective, one should not be
too optimistic as regards the chances of controlling viral
spread.

In some regions an effective vaccination against AD of
cattle that are in close proximity to swine has become desirable. Disappointing results in this respect, however, were
reported with an inactivated vaccine. Nevertheless, as the
challenge doses employed were rather high further research in
this direction (inactivated vaccines in cattle) appears
justified.

In the section 'Latent infection' it was shown that it is a
characteristic of herpes viruses to cause latent infection, and
ADV also has this effect. The presence of viral DNA has been
demonstrated by *in situ* cytohybridisation and DNA-DNA reassociation kinetics in the neural tissues of pigs in preliminary experiments for at least 13 weeks after infection. However, latent infection lasts considerably longer since ADV
could be detected by co-cultivation methods and after immunosuppression for at least 15 months after infection, and in pigs
which had been vaccinated with inactivated vaccine and thereafter infected with ADV, latent virus could be activated by
immunosuppression after $6\frac{1}{2}$ months.

Furthermore, it was shown that clinical symptoms of AD can
be evoked in latently infected pigs by immunosuppression $9\frac{1}{2}$
months after infection. Those animals also shed virus in their
nasal secretion, and virus could be isolated from the CNS and
the lungs with some of the killed animals.

The occurrence of latency of ADV in recovered and vaccinated infected pigs is of great importance for epizootiology and
control of AD. Further investigations are necessary to check
if latency in vaccinated animals is as strong and lasts as long
as in non-vaccinated animals. Furthermore, the distribution of

latently infected pigs in infected and vaccinated areas should
be examined. Besides, ADV latency is a model for other herpes
virus, especially herpes simplex virus, because with ADV one
can work in the natural host.

In the section 'Epidemiology, control and eradication'
epizootiological studies regarding AD were reported from 6 of
the member countries. They showed differences in occurrence
and prevalence of AD between the countries, but also within
the countries differences are found in the form of areas of
high or low prevalence of the disease. Total absence of AD is
found in some areas.

There is evidence of increasing problems and economic
losses caused by AD. This evolution should be seen in the
light of the establishment of larger intensive pig production
units and the appearance of virus strains with a higher pathogenicity than previously known. The laboratory findings seem
to reflect these differences in pathogenicity as syncytia-
forming isolates of the virus seem to possess a generally
higher pathogenicity for swine and cattle than non-syncytia-
forming strains.

Avoidance of contact with animals from uncontrolled herds
is considered to be the main factor in keeping herds free from
AD. Spread of AD through insects, birds or rodents does not
seem to be very likely, but observations from cases of respiratory infection in cattle and from outbreaks in closed herds
in the neighbourhood of large infected fattening pig units
indicate that air-borne transmission over short distances is a
factor which must be seriously considered. Experimental findings reported at the seminar indicate that wild swine may serve
as a reservoir for the infection.

Disease control by vaccination with inactivated and with
live vaccines was reported to be largely successful in controlling clinical outbreaks. However, one must be aware that vaccination does not prevent the spread of virus. The question of
using inactivated vaccines or live vaccines is a scientific and
a political problem. In some countries the use of live vaccines
is forbidden, whereas other countries use live vaccines on a
large scale.

Some countries have implemented legislative measures with the aim of controlling AD, and it could be recommended that areas with low prevalence of AD should establish eradication programmes, as eradication, if possible, seems to be the only way to control the disease in a satisfactory manner.

Whilst it seems desirable for minimal legislative requirements for the control of AD to be developed in the EC no conclusions were attempted by the participants of the scientific seminar. Veterinary authorities must be left to use the results of scientific work to prepare any appropriate legislation. To this end another meeting involving scientists and members of the veterinary authorities might well be most useful coordination in the near future.

LIST OF PARTICIPANTS

BELGIUM

Dr. P. Biront
Nationaal Instituut voor
  Diergeneeskundig Onderzoek
Groeselenberg 99
B-1180 Brussels

Dr. F. Castrijck
Provinciaal Laboratorium voor
  veeziektenbestrijding
Industrielaan 1
B-8100 Torhour

Dr. M. Pensaert
Fakulteit Diergeneeskunde
Laboratorium voor virologie
Casinoplein 24
B-9000 Ghent

DENMARK

Dr. J.B. Andersen
The Veterinary Directorate
21 Frederiksgade
DK-1265 Copenhagen K

Dr. V. Bitsch
State Veterinary Serum Laboratory
27 Bulöwsvej
DK-1870 Copenhagen V

Dr. K. Dalsgaard
State Veterinary Institute for
  Virus Research
Lindholm
DK-4771 Kalvehave

FEDERAL REPUBLIC OF GERMANY

Dr. R. Ahl
Bundesforschungsanstalt für
  Viruskrankheiten der Tiere
Paul-Ehrlich-Strasse 28
D-7400 Tübingen 1

Dr. P.C. Döller
Bundesforschungsanstalt für
  Viruskrankheiten der Tiere
Paul-Ehrlich-Strasse 28
D-7400 Tübingen 1

Dr. R. Franze
Bundesforschungsanstalt für
  Viruskrankheiten der Tiere
Paul-Ehrlich-Strasse 28
D-7400 Tübingen 1

Dr. B. Liess
Tierärztliche Hochschule
Institut für Virologie
Bischofsholer Damm 15
D-3000 Hanover

Dr. R.J. Lorenz
Bundesforschungsanstalt für
  Viruskrankheiten der Tiere
Paul-Ehrlich-Strasse 28
D-7400 Tübingen 1

Dr. H. Ludwig
Freie Universität Berlin
Fachbereich Veterinärmedizin
Institut für Virologie
Nordufer 20
  (im Robert Koch-Institut)
D-1000 Berlin 65

Dr. H. Mehrkens
Niedersächsisches Landes-
  verwaltungsamt
Tierseuchenkasse
Hildesheimer Strasse 82
D-3000 Hanover 1

Dr. V. Moennig
Tierärztliche Hochschule
Institut für Virologie
Bischofsholer Damm 15
D-3000 Hanover

Dr. V. Ohlinger
Bundesforschungsanstalt für
  Viruskrankheiten der Tiere
Paul-Ehrlich-Strasse 28
D-7400 Tübingen 1

Dr. G. Pauli
Freie Universität Berlin
Fachbereich Veterinärmedizin
Institut für Virologie
Nordufer 20
  (im Robert Koch-Institut)
D-1000 Berlin 65

Dr. H. Pittler
Bundesministerium für Ernährung
Landwirtschaft und Forsten
Rochusstrasse 1
D-5300 Bonn 1

Dr. H.-J. Rziha
Bundesforschungsanstalt für
  Viruskrankheiten der Tiere
Paul-Ehrlich-Strasse 28
D-7400 Tübingen 1

Dr. W. Schwöbel
Bundesforschungsanstalt für
  Viruskrankheiten der Tiere
Paul-Ehrlich-Strasse 28
D-7400 Tübingen 1

Dr. Sendbet
Tierärztliche Hochschule
Institut für Virologie
Bischofsholer Damm 15
D-3000 Hanover

Dr. O.C. Straub
Bundesforschungsanstalt für
  Viruskrankheiten der Tiere
Paul-Ehrlich-Strasse 28
D-7400 Tübingen 1

Dr. G. Wittmann
Bundesforschungsanstalt für
  Viruskrankheiten der Tiere
Paul-Ehrlich-Strasse 28
D-7400 Tübingen

FRANCE

Dr. J. Asso
Institut National de la Recherche
  Agronomique
F-78850 Thiverval-Grignon

Dr. B. Toma
Ecole Nationale Vétérinaire
7 avenue du Général de Gaulle
F-94704 Maisons-Alfort Cedex

Dr. P. Vannier
Station de Pathologie Porcine
B.P. no 9
F-22440 Ploufragan

GREECE

Dr. Brovas
Institute of Foot and Mouth
  Disease Research
Aghia Paraskevi
Attikis

IRELAND

Dr. P.J. O'Connor
Veterinary Laboratory
Abbotstown
Castleknock
Co. Dublin

Dr. P. Lenihan
Veterinary Laboratory
Abbotstown
Castleknock
Co. Dublin

ITALY

Dr. F. Cancellotti
Istituto Zooprofilattico
  Sperimentale delle Venezia
Via Orus, 2
I-35100 Padua

Dr. F. De Simone
Istituto Zooprofilattico
  della Lombardia e dell'Emilia
Via Bianchi, 7
I-25100 Brescia

Dr. F. Tozzini
Università di Pisa
Facoltà di Medicina Veterinaria
Istituto di Malattie Infettive
Viale delle Piagge, 2
I-56100 Pisa

Dr. Vivoli
Istituto Zooprofilattico
  dell'Umbria e delle Marche
Via Salvemini, 1
I-06100 Perugia

NETHERLANDS

Dr. A.L.J. Gielkens
The Central Veterinary Institute
Houtribweg 39
8221 RA Lelystad

Dr. P.W. de Leeuw
The Central Veterinary Institute
Houtribweg 39
8221 RA Lelystad

Dr. J.Th. van Oirschot
The Central Veterinary Institute
Houtribweg 39
8221 RA Lelystad

Dr. C. Terpstra
The Central Veterinary Institute
Houtribweg 39
8221 RA Lelystad

UNITED KINGDOM

Dr. A. Baskerville
Public Health Laboratory Service
Porton Down
Salisbury
Wiltshire
SP4 0JG

Dr. S.F. Cartwright
Ministry of Agriculture, Fisheries
  & Food
Central Veterinary Laboratory
New Haw
Weybridge
Surrey
KT15 3NB

Dr. R. Gaskell
University of Bristol
Department of Veterinary Medicine
Langford House
Langford
Bristol
BS18 7DU

Dr. S.A. Hall
Ministry of Agriculture, Fisheries
  & Food
Horseferry Road
London SW1P 2AE

Dr. J.B. McFerran
Veterinary Research Laboratories
Stormont
Belfast
BT4 3SD

Dr. E.N. Wood
Veterinary Investigation Centre
Government Buildings
Jupiter Road
Norwich
NR6 6ST

CEC

Dr. R. Masia

Dr. J. Connell